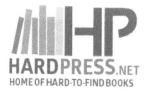

HARDPRESS.NET
HOME OF HARD-TO-FIND BOOKS

The Gentleman's Stable Directory
by William Taplin

Address:
HardPress
8345 NW 66TH ST #2561
MIAMI FL 33166-2626
USA
Email: info@hardpress.net

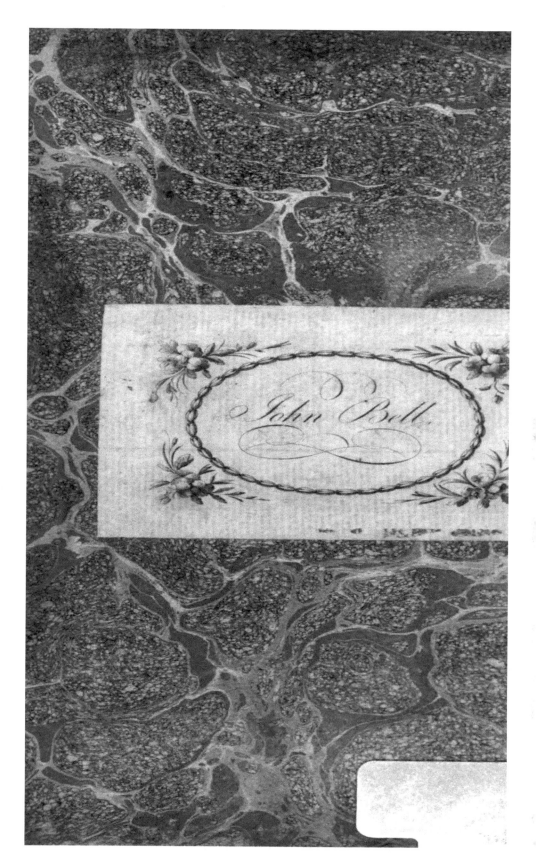

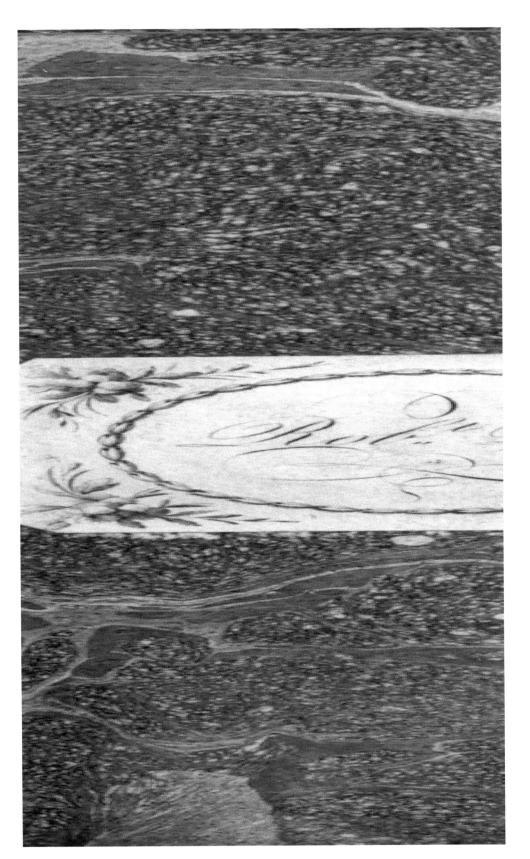

1897 e 138

The Third Edition, carefully corrected:

THE
GENTLEMAN's
STABLE DIRECTORY;

OR,

Modern System of Farriery.

VOLUME THE SECOND.

CONTAINING

EXPERIMENTAL REMARKS

UPON

BREEDING, STABLING,
BREAKING, EXERCISE, And
SHOEING, ROWELLING.

TO WHICH ARE ADDED,

PARTICULAR INSTRUCTIONS FOR THE
GENERAL MANAGEMENT OF

Hunters and Road Horses;

WITH

Concluding OBSERVATIONS upon the present
STATE of the TURF.

By WILLIAM TAPLIN.

LONDON:

Printed for G. G. J. and J. ROBINSON, Pater-noster-Row;
and C. and G. KEARSLEY, Fleet-street. 1793.

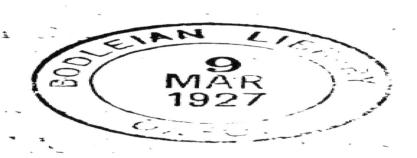

INTRODUCTION.

AFTER the many publications upon equeſtrian ſubjects, it may appear to ſome rather extraordinary that matter either *new*, *inſtructive*, or *entertaining*, can be produced to excite the ſerious attention even of thoſe, who are the moſt curious in their particular ſtuds and different appropriations; but ſuch admiration will as readily ſubſide, upon a retroſpective alluſion to the original motives of the various writers, the almoſt unlimited extent of the ſubject, the conſtantly encreaſing eſtimation of the object treated on, and the conſignment to

perpetual

perpetual allision of many literary productions, (unfortunately for their authors) fo
foon as they were brought to the teft of
public inveftigation.

The Gentleman's Stable Directory, having by the unprecedented rapidity of its
circulation through *ten large editions,* and
the acknowledged utility of its inftructions;
in a great degree fuperfeded former opinions, and eftablifhed the profeffional reputation of the writer; it will be hardly confidered a mark of prefumption, that (under
the flattering influence of popularity) the
fame pen fhould *once more* afpire to the hope
of applaufe, in his defire to extend the fyftem of management to a degree of confiftency hitherto undefcribed by any one of the
numerous authors, who have preceded us
upon the fame or fimilar fubjects.

So

So far as HEALTH and CONDITION are preferable to *difeafe*, fo much more defirable muft PREVENTION ever prove to the neceffity of *cure*. The purport of the prefent undertaking will, therefore, be found appertaining much more to fuch parts of ftabularian difcipline, as come under the diftinction of NOVELTY, and not treated on in a *direct way*, than at all applicable to the inveftigation or cure of difeafe; unlefs in occafional allufions or medical references evidently branching from the fubject, and tending to corroborate and improve the intentional uniformity of the whole. It being the predominant wifh of the writer, to render this publication fuch kind of collateral appendage to THE STABLE DIREC-TORY, as may conftitute *in both*, a complete chain of ufeful and entertaining inftruction for the improvement of the fpe-

cies

cies; their management in *ficknefs* or *health,* the *field* or *ftable,* including, under diftinct heads, fuch *facts* from *experience* and *infer—ences* from *nature,* as will, the author is earneftly induced to hope, procure him the approbation of thofe, by the fanction of whofe extenfive patronage he has been already fo very highly honoured.

THE

THE

MODERN SYSTEM

OF

FARRIERY.

BREEDING,

FROM its general magnitude, prevalent fashion, and great utility, is certainly entitled to precede every other subject, upon which we shall have occasion to enlarge, in the course of the work before us; and will afford ample opportunity to introduce such remarks and instructions, as may evidently tend to improve what is now become so universal, that the world at large, either in *pleasure, agriculture,* or *commerce,* seem interested in its success. Previous to embarkation in so extensive a field for investigation, it may be applicable to observe, that whatever *opinions* may be promulgated as matters of *recommendation,* they are not

to be confidered the delufive effect of fpeculative rumination, but the refult of long
perfonal experience and attentive obfervation
among horfes in my own poffeffion, from
brood mares and colts to every defcription,
whether for the *Turf, Field, Road, or Draft.*

Although fome of the fubjects upon which
we proceed to treat, may have been flightly mentioned by writers who have gone before us, it is generally known to have been
in fo fuperficial and unconnected a way,
that little information or inftruction could
be at all gleaned from their endeavours; a
few loofe hints upon each having been di-
greffively obtruded, or indifcriminately introduced, amidft topics to which they did
not bear the leaft allufion, and from whence
conclufions of the fmalleft utility could never be drawn.

Thefe errors it has been the principal defign to correct, by reducing to *diftinct heads*
all fuch obfervations and remarks as conftitute the body of the work, and are intended
as incentives to general improvement upon
the great variety of fubjects we fhall endeavour

deavour to contract into one *regular* and *uniform* point of view, with as little reference to, or animadverfion upon others, as the nature of fuch publication will admit.

So much has been faid upon the origin, inveftigation and cure of difeafe, in our former volume of *The Stable Directory*, that we fhall advert as little as poffible to medical confiderations; unlefs where from new occafions, or recent difcoveries, they become intimately and unavoidably connected with the fubject under difcuffion, as will probably prove the cafe with fome few heads, before we arrive at the goal of our undertaking.

BREEDING, though a fubject of palpable importance to the improvement of this moft ufeful animal, feems to have received lefs affiftance from literary exertion than any other that has ever attracted the time or attention of thofe naturalifts, who have in *other respects* contributed largely to the advantage and entertainment of the public. This affertion, generally confidered, has one ftriking exception in the peculiar and con-

ftantly

ftantly encreafing circumfpection, to improve (if poffible) what abfolutely appears to have already reached the very fummit of perfection: It will be readily conceived I allude to the almoft incredible care and attention beftowed upon the breed and management of our *blood horfes* for the turf, at this moment efteemed equal (if not fuperior) in *fpeed, bottom,* and difcipline to any other in the known world, particularly fince the fafhionable rage for *Arabians* has fo gradually declined.

Perfonal emulation amongft fome of the firft characters in the three kingdoms for near a century paft (with the moft unremitting perfeverance and practical experience of the fubordinate claffes, upon the advantageous croffes in *blood, bone, fhape, make,* and *ftrength)* has rendered NEWMARKET not only the firft feat of Equeftrian celebrity, but to a *breeder* and *fportfman,* one of the moft enchanting fcenes the univerfe has to produce. This part of the fpecies having, under fuch accumulated power and induftry, attained the very pinnacle of pre-eminence, nothing can be introduced to

breeders

breeders of such nice diftinction, that will poffibly add weight, or give force to fo complete a fyftem of unfullied perfection : As it is, however, generally admitted this fyftematic knowledge is by no means univerfal, fuch ufeful remarks and appertaining obfervations will be occafionally introduced under this head, as will afford ufeful intelligence or inftruction to thofe who have commenced breeders, without adverting to the qualifications or advantages abfolutely requifite for the fuccefsful management of a breeding ftud.

Taking leave for the prefent of *blood, pedigree,* and *fafhion,* we advert to the very capital breed of real Englifh hunters, and beautiful draft or carriage horfes, for which the counties of *York, Leicefter, Lincoln,* and *Northampton* are fo defervedly famous; they are certainly entitled to take the lead of every other county in the kingdom, not more in the care and fuperiority of their breed, than the confiftency of their proceedings to improve it. This preference, fo generally known and univerfally admitted, will create no furprife when we recollect

how

how admirably gifted by nature those counties are with requisite advantages, that other parts of England have not to boast; nor can they, from locality of situation, ever obtain.

Situate as the inhabitants are for these conveniences, they have consequently dedicated more time and attention to the improvement of the species in general, for the purposes of emolument, than the natives of most other counties, where the attempt (however judiciously made) becomes in some degree abortive, not only in respect to the deceptive expectation of profit, but a certain degeneracy from such *heterogeneous unions* (if I may be allowed the expression) as will be hereafter more clearly explained.

Customs and opinions upon this subject are both local and numerous, notwithstanding which they are frequently subservient to exigence of circumstances, and become productive of a propagation calculated for little more than a consumption of food, without a single prominent or distinguishing mark of blood, strength, or utility.

There

There are many substantial reasons to be adduced, why the breeders of the northern counties exceed all other parts of England, in the *consistency, strength, fashion*, and *symmetry* of their stock; for exclusive of their natural advantages of the most luxuriant pasture, and temperate climate for such purpose, they are rigidly attentive to every component minutiæ of the whole; not only to the shape, make, bone, strength, and uniformity of both *sire* and *dam*, but likewise to hereditary defects, blemishes, and deformities, rejecting every probability of *stain* or injury, divested of the paltry penurious considerations by which the conduct of many are regulated, who have been breeding *all their lives*, without the satisfaction of having ever *once* had a horse or mare of figure, fashion, or value in their possession.

This is a fact so clearly established, it will come home to the remembrance of every reader, when taking a *mental* survey of his rural neighbours, amongst whom he will perfectly recollect some *one or more* so invincibly attached to the merits of a *blind stallion*, or the virtues of his own *spider-legged mare*,

mare, that deftitute of judgment, and deaf to remonftrance, he ranks *(in imagination)* the produce *a prodigy* even *in embryo*, and proceeds regularly, year after year, encreafing the number, without a fingle addition to the improvement of the fpecies.

Thefe are the kind of *hypothetical* breeders, (and great plenty there are) who calculate doubly in error, by calculating upon *profit*, without a fingle contingent reflection upon *lofs*; ridiculoufly fuppofing a mare in foal, or after delivery, can fupport her own frame, and that of her offspring, upon *lefs food* than any other horfe or mare in conftant work; and begin breeding under an idea that it will be attended with little or no expence: Thus totally inadequate (or indifferent) to the generating of *flefh*, *blood*, and *bone* by the effect of nutrition, they penurioufly and inhumanly adopt a kind of temporary poverty, and after a year or two of artificial famine feem greatly furprifed, that *air* and *exercife* alone have not produced a colt, or filly, of equal *fize*, *ftrength*, and *perfection*, with thofe who have omitted no one expenfe or neceffary acquifition, that could in the leaft contribute to the formation of points so very desirable, in objects of such tedious expectation, and no little anxiety, before their merits or deficiencies could be at all satisfactorily ascertained. To avoid the accusation or even suspicion of intentional repetition, the uninformed reader is referred for an investigation of *nutriment*, its process and effects, to Vol. I. of the STABLE DIRECTORY, under the articles of *feeding*, *surfeit*, and *mange*, where he may collect every information he can possibly require upon the subject.

Those who succeed best, and render the business of breeding a matter of emolument, are evidently *gentlemen*, *graziers* or *farmers*, who adhere closely to the plan of producing a distinct stock for either the *turf*, *field*,] or *draft*, by a direct systematic union of the requisite qualifications in both *sire* and *dam*, without falling into the erroneous opinion of forming an *excellent hunter* from a blood horse and cart mare ; with similar changes eternally ringing by those who fall into the egregious mistake, of expecting that an equal partition of qualities from both sire and dam, will be so critically blended, as to
constitute

conftitute a medium *exactly between both,*
when every judicious obferver will be enabled to corroborate the opinion, that the
event frequently proves the error and de-
monftrates a palpable degeneracy from even
the *worft of the two.*

Thefe are the kinds of connection I have
before termed heterogeneous, upon experimental conviction, in fuch propagation; the
natural fluggifhnefs and inactivity of the old
Englifh draft horfe, whether it be in *fire* or
dam, generally predominates in the offspring, conftituting an object of difappointment where fo much improvement was expected by the crofs. I believe (without adverting to memory) that in a number of
years paft, I may boldly venture to affirm, I
could number at leaft twenty within the extenfive circle of my own acquaintance, who
full of expectation, and certain of fuccefs,
(in oppofition to every perfuafion) pofitively believed they fhould produce ftrong boney hunters of figure, fafhion, fpeed, and
ftrength in this way, when TIME, the ex-
pofitor of all doubts, has at length reduced
the conjecture to a certainty; and after waiting

ing four or five years for the fruit of their expectation to attain perfection, the *prodigy* has been unavoidably doomed to the drudgery of a butcher's tray, or the market cart of some industrious mechanic.

To this description of breeders, who are continually promoting the propagation of the species, without a single consistent idea, or relative consideration to the necessary requisites of *country* and *keep*, or qualifications of *fire* and *dam*, (with an additional prepossession in favour of certain ridiculous crosses) are we indebted for the infinity of horses annually produced in almost every (*improper*) part of the kingdom, that from want of shape, make, bone, fize, and strength are of no proportional value to the expense they have occasioned; they can pass under no distinct denomination, are applicable to no particular purpose, but become an expensive burden to the owners, who, too frequently fond of their own production, fix an imaginary value upon their *imperfections*, and year after year permit them to consume food and fodder that might evidently be appropriated

priated to fervices of much greater public utility and private emolument.

To the conftant increafe of horfes that are of *little or no value,* may be attributed, in a collateral degree, the alarming advance in almoft every neceffary of life where the indigent and neceffitous are moftly interefted without exception : But as the introduction of minute calculations to demonftrate the fact, would be digreffing from the fubject before us, I fhall only refer the attention of the curious reader for a moment, to a comparative reflection upon the incredible confumption of pafturage in fummer, and corn with hay in winter, that might through *other channels* be much more adapted to the promotion of a general good.

After the remarks hitherto introduced upon the inconfiftency and very *fafhionable abfurdity,* of even attempting to breed horfes in fuch parts of the kingdom as are but ill adapted to the purpofe, whether from the hilly ftate of the country, the infertility of the foil, want of luxuriance in the pafture, or many other concomitant obftacles, (totally

unat-

unattended to by the parties concerned) it becomes perfectly applicable, to revert once more to the frequent and inconsiderate practice of uniting horses and mares, with every joint hereditary blemish or defect that can render the offspring unpromising; without a single perfection, or encouraging ray of expectation, to constitute a junction of points, possibly tending in the least to form *a produce* even tolerably adequate to the particular purpose for which it may be intended when at a proper age it is brought into use. *Such breeders* seldom pay the least attention to *merits, tempers, vices, constitutional blemishes,* or hereditary defects of either sire or dam; the grand and leading object is, to obtain a horse or mare of their " *own breed:* " in that happy thought alone is to consist their perfection, and in such expanded idea is buried every just or relative consideration.

Predominant reasons are by no means wanting to elucidate this strange and invincible infatuation; for penury in some, absolute inadvertency in others, and palpable indolence in the remaining class, effect the
annual

annual increase to a certainty; the same unaccountable prejudice that prompts them to
commence breeders, without a consistent
qualification in *horse* or *mare*, influences
them also to reserve a colt of such breed to
perform the office of STALLION, in the vicinity of their own residence, that the ab-
surdity began by themselves may be persevered in by others: This *prodigy*, with all
his imperfections, is permitted to cover *gratis*, or for a trifling pecuniary consideration
to the servant, (as a complete gratification
of the owner's ambition in breeding) and
proving a local convenience, is readily em-
braced by the inactive classes before described, while others of more *prudence, spirit,
emulation*, or consistency of conduct, will rather send a mare fifty miles, and encounter
any consequent expense, to obtain a horse
whose shape, make, bone, strength, and action are calculated to correspond with the
dam, promising to produce a colt or filly,
adequate in figure and value to the purpose
originally intended.

Notwithstanding these necessary precautions, the long standing adage of there being

ing "no one rule without an exception," is sometimes verified; and this even in the first *blood studs* in the kingdom, where the strictest attention to every confonant point is so rigidly persevered in, that the least deviation from symmetry, speed and perfection could hardly be believed, did not the result so clearly demonstrate the frequency of the fact.

Extraordinary as such circumstance may appear, it is certainly true that many of the most capital runners, when they have become stallions, seldom or ever begot a winner, though the mares have been selected with the greatest care as objects of equal perfection. These remain among the abstruse recesses of nature that will, perhaps, ever continue unexplained; we may therefore patiently adopt a supposition as a substitute for difcovery, presuming, " so far shall ye go, and no farther," is all that can be advanced in elucidation of the subject.

In corroboration of this well-authenticated assertion, great numbers might be particularized of the present day, where the progeny

progeny have degenerated in almoft every point from fire and dam; but the rapid fucceffion of one capital horfe upon another, (feafon after feafon) would render the names of fuch as might *now be mentioned*, a matter of oblivion to future readers, and prove to them little or nothing of an opinion we wifh to eftablifh beyond the power of contradiction.

So much chance appertains to the act of breeding for the Turf, that *one lucky get* very frequently conftitutes a STALLION of FASHION, to which the rage of future feafons becomes incredibly fubfervient; innumerable inftances might be quoted in proof of this fporting credulity, but we will contract the number to fuch only as are too eminent in their ftock ever to be forgotten, fo long as the pedigrees of "great, great, great, great, great grand dams and grand-fires" fhall be tranfmitted to pofterity.

It is now within the memory of hundreds upon the turf, that old *Marfk* (a moft capital runner of his time) covered in Windfor Foreft and its neighbourhood, a very great number of mares fo low as half a guinea

guinea each, but upon the production of ECLIPSE, (a horfe whofe almoft unprecedented qualifications and performances will in all probability never be forgotten) his price was enhanced to fifty guineas, and that only for a certain number in the feafon, out of which (though much advanced in years) he produced many winners, when the felection of mares became fo much in his favour.

Such fluctuation of popularity ftill depends upon the uncertainty of events, an additional proof of which deferves to be recorded as worthy the attention of fportfmen to whom it is not very generally known, though too well authenticated to admit even a fhadow of doubt, and reduces to a certainty the former obfervation, that CHANCE alone is often entitled to the merit fo conftantly attributed to *judgment* and *penetration.*

The dam of *Eclipfe* having been covered in that feafon by both SHAKESPEARE and MARSK, it remained a matter of doubt for fome days with his late Royal Highnefs the Duke of Cumberland and his ftud groom, to *which* the colt should be ascribed; however, the time of the mare's bringing forth (during the great Eclipse) coming nearest to the day she was booked to have been covered *by Marsk*, to him was attributed the distinguished honour of getting one of the first horses in the known world; whose strength, power and speed were so great, that he with ease *double-diftanced* the most capital horses when running with twelve stone for the king's plate, and afterwards *walked over* most of the king's plate courses in the kingdom. The doubt respecting his *fire* having been thus removed, with at least an apparent degree of precision, it may naturally be supposed to have been decided with the strictest justice; but had such doubt still existed upon his own pedigree, the *superiority* of his qualifications would have appeared in his produce, he having proved the fire of a most wonderful progeny in *Mercury, Meteor, Soldier, Gunpowder, King Fergus, Dungannon, Bowdrow, Jupiter, Vertumnus,* and many others too numerous to recite, whose blood (in so great a variety of branches) will no doubt be

continued

continued with fashionable crosses to the end of time.

It is hardly possible for one little acquainted with the customs and manners of the turf to conceive, how the decision of a single match or sweepstakes alters the properties and value of a stallion, whose reputation is placed (in blood and performance) upon the summit of eminence; for should some of the first of his get that start fortunately become winners, such circumstance instantly enhances his superiority to a degree of enthusiasm, and more business being marked out for him in the act of pro-creation than nature is equal to, his number of mares are consequently limitted, and he becomes immediately an object of great annual emolument, several instances having occurred in the last twenty years, where different stallions have produced to their owners five and twenty hundred pounds *in one season*.

But in this state of acknowledged excellence and superiority, they are still subject to the versatility of chance, and one " unlucky step for ever *damns their fame*;"

for

for two or three of his get being beat at a subfequent Newmarket meeting, the victorious fire foon fuperfedes the favourite, who, falling into the back ground of the picture, glides imperceptibly to an almoft total oblivion. In fuch fluctuation or fucceffion, fubmits the fame of an *Herod* to an *Eclipfe*, an *Evergreen* to a *Sweetbriar*, and a very long lift of etceteras to thofe reigning favourites of the prefent day *Highflyer* and *Woodpecker*, the former of which having produced thirty-nine winners of ninety-one capital prizes, and the latter feventeen winners of fifty-four, both in the year 1789 only, it will create no furprife that they at prefent enjoy, under the funfhine of popular influence, a more extenfive and beautiful *feraglio* than any Arabian on earth has ever had to boaft.

Having ventured a few remarks upon what I before termed exceptions to general rules, or predominant opinions, it becomes perfectly confiftent to ftrengthen a belief of fuch poffibilities, by the recital of a direct contraft within my own knowledge and perfect remembrance, of a galloway that never

ver

ver exceeded *thirteen* hands, though got by *Marſk,* (who was a large horſe) out of a full ſized hackney mare in the neighbourhood of Windſor; as well as a very large, boney, handſome uſeful gelding full fifteen hands, out of *a poney mare* under *twelve,* that was bought of a troop of gipſies near Baſingſtoke for a ſingle guinea. An encreaſed liſt of ſuch inſtances might be eaſily formed and equally authenticated; but theſe are ſufficient to encounter the aſſertions of thoſe who *ſeem* firmly to believe the impracticability of obtaining *bone, ſize,* or *ſtrength,* but from horſes and mares of ſuch ſize and bone only; and although it is certainly right to admit the probability of deviation from ſire and dam in ſuch caſes, yet the minute inveſtigation of cauſes muſt lead us into a field of phyſical reaſoning, and anatomical diſquiſition, that would prove in general reading too remote and extenſive for the ſubject before us.

There are, however, very juſt and fair reaſons to be adduced, why theſe contraſts ſo frequently occur in oppoſition to the eſtabliſhed notions of breeding, without at all

C 3

advert-

adverting to an abstrufe animadverfion upon the "animalculæ in femine mafculino," the probable expanfion or contraction of the uterus, the act of generation, the crifis of conception, the formation and growth of the fœtus in embryo, with other relative confiderations that might very well bear ferious and fcientific invefigation, were we at all inclined to *perplex* by the introduction of conjectures calculated to promote the learned lucubrations of a certain fociety, but little to entertain the members of a fporting club at Newmarket, or to improve the different gradations of their numerous dependents.

The uncertainty of all human expectations being therefore univerfally admitted, and fuch matters of *opinion only* paffed over as can never be brought to the decifive teft of infallibility; it is natural to conclude (notwithftanding fuch cafual deviations) much more may be expected in the produce, from a direct coincidence of parts with an union of ftrength, fhape and fymmetry, than from any improper or convenient connection founded only upon the *local fituation* of fire

and

and dam, without a single reference to their different natural blemishes, defects, imperfections, or hereditary taints, of which many may be frequently difcovered by care and the neceffary circumfpection.

After the introduction of fuch remarks as evidently tend to conftitute the neceffary apology for, and prelude to the undertaking, it will be naturally expected I fhould revert to inftructions that become immediately worthy the attention of every young and inexperienced breeder, who feels a defire to excel in his ftock from the motive of emulation, amufement or emolument. It has been before hinted, that thofe fucceed beft for either who propagate the different kinds according to the diftinct fpecies of each, whether for the *Turf*, *Field*, or *Draft*, without defcending to the adoption of croffes in themfelves erroneous and feldom productive.

In the prefent enormous price given for horfes of every denomination (univerfally faid and believed to be occafioned by the conftant and unprecedented exportation of our moft valuable Englifh breed) it is almoft difficult to decide, which clafs contributes moft to the profit of the breeder. I cannot, however, in my own opinion, hefitate a moment to pronounce the preference to have fallen upon thofe that turn the fooneft into fpecie : Of thefe, for inftance, are the beft bred *blood ftock*, now in the higheft and moft incredible ftate of cultivation ; the common marketable prices of thefe, if of the firft pedigrees, and brought to a promifing fize *when yearlings*, are one hundred and fifty guineas for *colts*, and one hundred for *fillies*, at which they pafs current, provided they are croffed in blood from any of the ftallions whofe celebrity we have before had occafion to mention.

Without enlarging upon this fort of fporting fpeculation, I fhall only obferve, that under certain regulations and very nice diftinction, with great care and unremitting attention, this may prove a much more profitable mode of breeding for thofe who wifh to afcertain a fixed emolument, (without hazarding the lofs of a certainty in *breaking, training, racing, &c.*) as is the prudent

practice

practice of the most eminent dealer in the kingdom, who is annually accumulating a very confiderable fortune by the conftant transfer of equeftrian property in its infancy, rather than encounter the incredible expence and anxiety of a ftud in training, the glorious uncertainty of the turf, the unbounded infolence of the neceffary dependents, and the *immaculate purity* of thofe to whom your honour and property muft be eventually entrufted, as will be more fully explained when the fubject comes again under confideration, towards the conclufion of the work.

Concluding, therefore, this clafs of breeders to derive the greateft pecuniary advantage from their increafe of ftock, by converting it expeditioufly into cafh with fo little trouble, expence, and inconvenience, it is not matter of furprife that the rage for blood and pedigree fhould be daily increafing, (and likely to continue fo) though the palpable effect of *" training on and training off,"* annually diffipates and reduces to humiliating indigence fome of the moft princely fortunes in this and the neighbouring kingdom

kingdom of Ireland, where the thirst for equestrian pre-eminence is *equal*, if not *superior* to our own.

The breed of horses most profitable to the graziers and breeders of Lincoln, Leicester, Northampton, and some few other counties, adapted by nature to the purpose, are probably the old English black draft horses, so remarkable for their bone, strength, and hardiness of constitution; These, from their great size, beauty and uniformity, become to every curious observer, objects of singular attraction; their wonderful power in business renders them in general request, and the breed is cultivated with the strictest attention to corresponding points and perfections in both sire and dam, little inferior to the class last treated on. STALLIONS of eminence in the above counties are estimated at very considerable sums, and frequently let out to cover from one hundred to two hundred guineas for the season; the stock generally come into gentle use at two years old, or under, and when brought to a good size in proper time, frequently fetch from thirty to fifty guineas at two and three years old.

Those

Those horses paffing under the denomination of *hunters*, but more particularly the common croffes for *roadfters* and *backs*, can by no means prove fo generally profitable, when all contingencies are taken into confideration; the length of time they are obliged to be kept on hand and maintained, (till at leaft four years old) with the unfavourable changes they may probably undergo before they can be brought to the ultimate market of emolument moft applicable to their different qualifications, render the whole a matter of much greater uncertainty than with horfes of the preceding defcription; for the unavoidable difficulties of cutting, breaking, backing, docking, and nicking, render them ferious operations, the fuccefs of which cannot be afcertained without encountering a chance of misfortune or failure to injure the fubject and affect his value.

Notwithftanding thefe confiderations are intended for general application, it muft be remembered they will ever remain fubject to the different degrees of fuccefs, arifing from the variety of circumftances already explained. Counties, as I have before remarked, differ

differ fo very much in their fituation and fertility for breeding, that many will not produce horfes of fize, and the defirable qualifications, at even *treble* their *real value*, when brought to the very higheft market for difpofal : For it is a fact indifputably certain, that nothing but a part of the kingdom remarkable for the abundance and luxuriance of its herbage, can ever produce ftock of fize and value to render breeding a matter of emolument; the attempt, therefore, in unfavourable fituations, muft ever recoil upon the adventurer with additional difappointment.

Thefe obfervations, fo immediately relative to the idea of profit and lofs, are by no means introduced to reftrain or deter thofe from the practice, who are fo unavoidably circumftanced *in fituation,* as to breed under fuch difadvantage from the motive of *amufement only,* where pecuniary compenfation is no way concerned or expected; it is, however, to be prefumed, that occafional references to the inftructions hereafter inculcated, upon an extenfive fcale for the improvement of ftock in general (without again

adverting

adverting to the fuperiority that one part of the country enjoys over another) may contribute more to a gratification of their wifhes, than to pay an implicit obedience to the effect of chance unaffifted by any perfonal effort " to better the example."

Previous to further difcuffion of the fubject before us, it is worthy admiration in how many ways the animal production of the temperate region we enjoy has been enabled to demonftrate its individual excellence over a fimilar part of the creation, when tranfported from any other part of the globe. This remark might be juftified by a very flight comparative view of the different animals, whofe abilities or power (according to their diftinct qualifications) have been purpofely placed in competition with others to prove the inferiority ; one, however, comes immediately applicable to our prefent defign. Attempts have been repeatedly made by very ftrenuous advocates of the firft eminence and property, to improve the breed of our own nation by the elaborate introduction and crofs of the moft celebrated ARABIANS, carefully felected under impor-

tant

tant commiffions, where expenfe and trouble proved only inferior confiderations : But the trial afforded by *time*, and experience by *obfervation*, have fully fhewn the improbability of adding to the perfections of the true Englifh blood horfes by the importation of theirs.

This rage for improvement with a crofs from the blood of Arabia, was near half a century paft very *fafhionably* predominant, but has fo gradually declined for the laft twenty years, that they are held in no kind of eftimation by any fyftematic fportfman or breeder in the kingdom. The original advantage expected in the crofs, was fome addition *in fpeed*, even to our fleeteft mares; this, when obtained, was totally counteracted by a want of *bottom*, for after repeated trials, the moft exact and difinterefted, they were found incapable of keeping *their rate* for much more than a mile, and confequently became of fo little confequence to a *racing ftud*, that a fhort time will, in all probability, render them of no other utility than to conftitute part of the retinue in the triumphant return of an *Englifh Nabob*, or an addition

tion to the *oftrich, porcupine,* and *rhinoceros* of fome eccentric collector of curiofities.

BRACKEN has introduced a few judicious remarks upon the fubject of breeding, but in his *ufual way* fo perpetually interfperfed with inapplicable ftories and ftrange conclufions, that you are dragged through forty or fifty pages of extraneous and digreffive matter to be informed, that " Spanking Roger, belonging to the late Sir Edmund Bacon, was a *round barrelled horfe* ;" " that Mr. William Penry cured his ftammering patients of that defect in fpeech by *purging* ; that " a mare belonging to Mr. T. Makin, of Prefcot, in Lancafhire, run with her fore feet as wide as *a barn door* ; yet fhe ran as faft as moft of her fize, which was all owing to bringing in her haunches quick, for " *they muft needs go when the devil drives* ;" that " an old woman can cure a wound as well as a furgeon ;" that " phyficians may, from their ignorance, be confidered a fet of *vile pick-pockets,* almoft as numerous as the *caterpillars of the law* ;" that " he who fails with a *bad wind* had need underftand tacking about ;" with a great number of *curious remarks,* equally fublime, and as highly

highly applicable to the subject he was treating on; upon which he has introduced, no new matter in any direct chain of connection, tending at all to enlighten the topic or improve the management, having literally taken up the busineſs by way of amuſement, and laid it down preciſely where he found it.

We might here, with great ſeeming propriety, introduce a long liſt of inſtructions, containing the ſhape, make, bone, ſtrength, with all the variety of points neceſſary (or at leaſt likely) in horſe and mare, to conſtitute a progeny of promiſing perfections; but thoſe requiſites are ſo extenſively and accurately deſcribed between the twelfth and twentieth pages of The Gentleman's Stable Directory, Vol. I. and muſt be ſo nicely implanted in the mind and memory of almoſt every ſportſman or breeder, that a repetition here might be candidly deemed entirely ſuperfluous, and conſequently render us ſubject to an accuſation we wiſh moſt attentively to avoid.

Such deſcription of points and qualifications

cations, ftanding therefore not only incontroverted, but in poffeffion of general acquiefcence, to *thofe pages* the juvenile or inexperienced enquirer is referred for any additional information he may wifh to obtain ; this reference being juftified only upon the natural prefumption, that there will be very few purchafers of the prefent work, but what are holders of the firft Volume of the Stable Directory likewife.

Having there fo extenfively fhewn what are the requifites defirable to obtain, we now proceed to explain what the defects are moft neceffary to be difcovered in either fire or dam, that the poffible retention of *hereditary taints, defects* or *deformities,* may be the better avoided ; for although it remains, and in all probability ever will, a matter of ambiguity why an unblemifhed horfe and mare may produce a colt or filly full of *difeafe* or *deformity,* it by no means follows that a difeafed or deformed fire and dam are equally likely to produce a progeny of perfection : This being unequivocally admitted, (as by every impartial inveftigator of nature it certainly muft be) it will undoubtedly prove

an act of confiftency to evade fo palpable a
chance of difappointment, by forming an union
of propriety apparently calculated (from every
external appearance) to tranfmit fuch original
purity to their produce.

To effect this, the mare having been obtained correfponding in fize, frame, bone,
and ftrength, with the wifh of the breeder,
and found upon accurate examination to be
perfectly free from the blemifhes and defects
fo frequently mentioned, the choice of a
ftallion becomes the object of ferious attention; in him fhould be accumulated all the
points and good qualities it is poffible for a
fingle object to poffefs, upon a proof exceeding all fpeculation, (and this every obfervant
naturalift will allow) that the produce, whether male or female, much more frequently
acquires and retains the fhape, make, marks,
and difpofition of the fire than the dam; and
although fuch affertion may not obtain immediate credit with many, yet rigid obfervation has long fince demonftrated the fact,
and juftifies the great confiftency of rejecting
ftallions with the leaft appearance of difeafe,
blemifh, or bodily defect, indicating even the
flighteft

flighteft probability of tranfmiffion to the offspring.

Suppofing a neighbouring *ftallion*, and fuch there generally is in every part of the kingdom, to have great recommendation in his favour, as to the matter of common enquiry and fafhionable figure, it is ftill neceffary to defcend to the minutiæ of fymmetry in *head, neck, fhoulder, forehand, ribs, back, loins, joints,* and *pafterns,* attending to a ftrict uniformity in the fhape, make, and texture of the *very hoofs,* and were it poffible (which in almoft every cafe it certainly is not) even to afcertain the temper and difpofition of both fire and dam, rather than be acceffary to a procreation of vices or imperfections, that by a more judicious election may be fo eafily avoided.

After all that can poffibly be written (and if it were probable THAT ALL could be univerfally read) upon this fubject, every reader poffeffing the power of free agency has ftill the privilege to reject any opinion not perfectly coincident with the plan he may have adopted, and to enjoy the uncon-

trolled

trolled right of perfevering in his own decifion; but prefuming on the tafk I have un-
dertaken, I confcientioufly recommend a proper examination to difcover the ftate of the
wind, fpavins, curbs, tendency to cracks or
greafe, bad conformation of the *feet,* as corns,
thrufh, or long and narrow heeled hoofs, either of all which, would furnifh fufficient
foundation to prejudice me againft him as a
fire, however well I might be pleafed with
his other moft promifing perfections.

These cafual blemifhes or hereditary defects being carefully avoided, we come to an
enquiry of much greater confequence, the inattention to which has been productive of
more difappointment and vexation to the before-defcribed clafs of unthinking breeders,
than perhaps any other part of their inconfiftency. Oppofite opinions will always be the
fupport of two diftinct claffes, *the right and
the wrong;* for while one party afferts (from
experience and obfervation) the great hazard and certain danger of breeding from a
blind ftallion, the other, from innate obftinacy or affected fuperiority of penetration, is
determined to encounter fuch indifcretion
upon

upon the heroic bafis of " the more danger the more honour," and in the event repentantly difcover the want of knowledge and prudence in themfelves they fo exultingly prefume to arraign in doubting the judgment of others.

The introduction of new opinions as mere matter of *fpeculation*, is a communication of juft as much as amounts to *nothing* ; fuch conjectures, without the fhew of reafon to eftablifh an apparent difcovery of the *proof,* would be gaining no ground in the eftimation of public opinion, nor laying any juft claim to credit for the refponfibility of our affertions. Luckily, however, for the fupport of the fubject before us, *accumulated proofs* are by no means wanting (even within the pale of my own perfonal experience and conviction) to counteract oppofite opinions, whether imbibed from prejudice, obftinacy, or ignorance.

Adverting again to what I fo lately admitted, the *poffibility* of found fires and mares producing a defective progeny ; and, *vice verfa,* that *blind ftallions* may fometimes get colts

with

with good eyes; yet the chance, or rather, imprudence, of breeding from such had much better be avoided; as the incontrovertible evidence I shall introduce, upon the folly of embarking in such an expedition, (where the odds are entirely against the adventurer, without a single point in his favour) must prove exactly similar to playing at *hazard* with *false dice,* where you may *eternally* lose, but never can rise a *winner.*

It is likely these considerations may want proper weight with those who display a contemptuous smile of disbelief at the very idea of transmitting hereditary blemishes or defects from sire to son, as the result of Cynical opposition to the *more rational* system they adopt of annually breeding under every possible disadvantage, in confirmation of their inexperience: I shall therefore recommend to their *incredulity* a few instances, confirming as *facts* what may have been hitherto considered matters of doubt, without the least criterion for general decision.

The first opportunity I could avail myself of to justify or render nugatory my opinion of

the

the impropriety and danger of breeding from
horfes of this defcription, was in the year
1773 or 1774, when a great number of
mares in that neighbourhood had been covered by a very popular "*blind ftallion*," (for
that was really the appellation under which
he paffed) of the Hon. T. King's, near
Ripley, in Surrey, whofe pedigree, fhape,
make, figure, and qualifications, were fo effectually fafcinating with the multitude, that
the want of *eyes* did not feem at all to im-
pede the daily progrefs of his procreation.
The infection of fafhion was then (and ever
will be) as predominant as at prefent ; for the
flaves to that *gew-gaw* continued to bring
their mares in unremitting rotation, and never difcovered their own *want of fight*, or
common comprehenfion, till the *third* or
fourth year, when the major part of the produce became as blind as the fire.

Still anxious to afcertain to fome ftate of
certainty, an object of fo much confequence
(not only to the fporting people, but the
world at large) as the hereditary tranfmiffion
of this defect, I was conftantly upon the
watch to enlarge my enquiries to fome de-

D 4 gree

gree of satisfaction; I remained, however, without any thing perfectly conclusive till the spring of the year 1780, when a grey horse called *Jerry Sneak*, (that had proved a tolerable runner, in the possession of LORD SPENCER HAMILTON) coming into my hands upon very easy terms just as his eyes were failing, I covered a few mares, *gratis*, with him in the neighbourhood of *Frimley*, near *Bagshot*, which having made memorandum of, with a design to purchase any of the produce that appeared tolerable promising, and making my excursion through the different parishes to obtain from the parties the necessary information, I found in the *fourth year* many of the produce *totally blind*, and the remainder nearly so without exception.

Facts (it is universally admitted) are stubborn things, and to the establishment of *this fact* I have been anxiously labouring as to the acquisition of individual emolument, though I have ever considered it a promotion of general good, in which the community is so much interested, that it would be an absolute want of philanthropy to con-

ceal

ceal whatever could in the leaft tend to an additional difcovery upon the fubject.

It is not the purport of the prefent work (nor is it at all applicable to the pur-pofe) to enter into phyfical refearches, lead-ing the reader through a long chain of phi-lofophical difquifition upon LEWENHOCK's microfcopic inveftigation of the *animalculæ* contained in the *femen* of animals, founding upon fuch enquiry a thoufand conjectures refpecting this abftrufe procefs of nature, that may very much perplex the mind, but can neither tend to entertain or improve the judgment.

Of as little confequence or advantage it muft certainly prove, to attempt any exact decifion by what nice and undifcovered ope-ration in the animal fyftem, a horfe is ren-dered firft *partially*, then *totally* blind by too frequent or hard racing; as well as the very common occurrence of a ftallion's becoming equally fo by too conftant and repeated *cover-ing*, though the act itfelf is a fpontaneous effort of nature.

However

However difficult it may be to furnifh an
opinion applicable to *every idea*, I believe
with the fcientific inveftigator there need be
little fcruple to hazard a profeffional defcription, by what means fo ferious a revolution
in the frame is effected; for the *brain* being
the very bafis of the nervous fyftem, and
the *nerves* the acknowledged feat of *pain* and
pleafure, any exquifite or preternatural extreme in either may be productive of great
debilitation, and the *optic nerves* being neareft the *origin*, may become more fenfibly
affected in a *paralytic* or fome other degree,
than any fubfequent pair, and the fight gradually decline from a partial vifion to total
blindnefs.

For the honor of human nature, I can
but moft earneftly wifh the applicable introduction of thefe remarks may induce the parties interefted in the event, to be in future
a little lefs ftrenuous in their different exertions, whether for credit or emolument; the
firft never to diftrefs one of the nobleft animals on earth, by thofe frequent and fevere
runnings that evidently exhauft nature to fuch
a ftate of mortification; or the latter in the
truly contemptible method of letting a horfe
cover

cover such an infinity of mares, as not uncommonly terminates in the irretrievable loss
of his eyes, but the inevitable loss of his reputation also, as " *a certain foal-getter* ;" for
the great number of mares covered by him
without produce, brings his character the following season into disrepute, should even the
state of his bodily strength, constitution, or
chance, preserve his eyes from the great probability of annihilation: This remark appertaining only to the owners of stallions who
attend the markets of different towns every
day in the week during the whole season,
exclusive of the additional portion of business in their own neighbourhood on the *Sunday morning*.

Of these there are so great a number, and
in their performance so general a failure, that
it is absolutely wonderful how so many can
become dupes to the customary infatuation,
of leading a mare to any market town, to
be served by a horse who is continually
covering from four or five, to eight or ten
mares in every twenty-four hours during the
season; with the additional consideration, that
these *extra exertions* are most frequently
made

made under the CORRUPT INFLUENCE of *ftimulants, provocatives*, and *cordials* adapted to the purpofe, and fuppofed to act with the fame excitement as *cantharides* upon the human body. Incredible as it may appear, (to thofe whofe fituation in life has rendered them little fubject to difcoveries of this kind) I have been repeatedly called upon in my profeffional department, to difpenfe large quantities of *this very article* to many of thofe who travel the country with ftallions of fuch denomination; firft obtaining from them a communication of the ufe it was intended for before they were entrufted with it, upon an experimental conviction of its danger; having in the courfe of my private medical practice known one life loft, and another miraculoufly faved, where it had been given under the denomination of *love powder* for the unfair gratification of the worft of purpofes.

Without entering again upon the act of generation, the femen, or animalculæ contained in it, as before adverted to, can any intelligent reader, to whofe deliberate attention thefe pages may become fubject, be at
all

all furprifed, that in fuch a conftrained and proftituted ftate of NATURE, fo few of her attempts fhould be productive of fuccefs ? . . . Here we might be readily induced to enter another large field for fcientific difquifition; but as it would evidently extend not only beyond the prefent purpofe, but prove " *cavier to the multitude,*" our inferior clafs of readers might occafionally exclaim with MUNGO in the PADLOCK, " What fignify *me read,* if me *no underftand !*"

Avoiding, therefore, the indifference in general fhewn to remote medical explanation, and dull anatomical defcriptive, I come directly to a queftion founded in reafon, upon the merits of which the interefted part of the world will be enabled to decide, at leaft fo far as correfponds with their own opinions upon the fubject. Can it be poffibly believed or expected (but by the moft illiterate, who, in fact, poffefs the grofs comforts of life *only,* and never enjoy the fublime gratification of *thinking,)* that horfes thus eternally jaded and harraffed, not only with the diurnal routine of copulation, but the inceffant fatigue of travelling perpetually, can be at all

equal

equal to the Herculean task assigned them?
Can it be matter of surprise, that not more
than one-third, or, upon a more favourable
computation, *one half at most*, of the mares
covered in this way produce a colt, and that
the half of those so produced, never come
to a proper size, bone, or strength; then can
there remain a doubt in the mind of any
unprejudiced man living, but to these causes
may be attributed some portion of that deficiency so generally complained of, and too
frequently attributed to the *want of bone* in
fire or dam?

Having hitherto introduced what I conceive to be the leading qualifications in horse
and mare, to render the business of breeding pleasant and advantageous, we come next
to consider the season most proper for bringing them together; as it must be admitted,
an inconvenience will certainly arise to the
mare by foaling too early in the spring,
or to the *produce* by falling too late in the
summer, it will undoubtedly prove more
eligible to adhere a little to the line of mediocrity, letting either extreme be carefully
avoided.

Never-

Nevertheless, it must be understood, this circumstance can by no means be altogether universal, as it depends in some measure upon the country and situation; the pasturage being of different states in different counties, and dependant upon the fertility of soil as well as the temperature of climate, the season is consequently forwarder, at least the herbage, (by a fortnight or three weeks) in one part of the kingdom than another, a circumstance that should always be properly attended to by the parties concerned.

It will therefore prove perfectly consistent in all counties, however they may be situated, to have the produce and pasture appearing at the same time as nearly as fluctuating or unavoidable circumstances will allow; for when mares are permitted to take the horse too soon in the season, they bring forth before there is sufficient grafs for their support, and being necessarily assisted with dry food, the lacteals, (or milk vessels) for want of gradual supply and expansion, become contracted; the very sharp winds early in the spring, with a restraint in food, sometimes so stints the colt, (particularly, should a

wet

wet unfavourable summer and severe winter follow) that he never reaches a proper size in growth, but displays the disadvantage of his earliest state when arrived at maturity.

It is no uncommon thing in different parts of the country, to observe mares that have dropped their foals early, (before there is a blade of grass for their support) placed in a rick yard, where, by incessantly *tugging* out a *scanty living*, it is ridiculously believed both mare and colt are indulging most lux-uriously, though the direct contrary is really the case; hay may undoubtedly (if admini-stered in due supplies) contribute a suffici-ency of support for the mare, but is not calculated to yield, even in almost constant mastication, any great nutritious superflux for the subsistence and desirable improve-ment of the colt. As there is a very great difference in the nutritive qualities of food, so is there a very material difference in the milk it produces; indifferent or sparing ali-ment will certainly produce a thin aqueous impoverished milk, of quality and in quan-tity to sustain and barely subsist nature, but by no means to give it *strength, vigour, growth,*

growth, or the formation of flesh and *bone* so generally defirable.

However haftily fome part of the world may be inclined to decide, (as every obferver has a right to indulge his own opinion) there can be no doubt but to the inconfiderate practice of inadvertently leaving mares and colts to fubfift upon *bare land,* or barren paftures, for the firft fummer, and a fucceffive fcene of poverty in the enfuing winter, are we in fome degree indebted for a proportion of thofe horfes I have before defcribed, as coming under no denomination, applicable to no particular purpofe, never rifing to any confiderable worth, and doing fo little credit to the breeder, that you can never difcover (if you were fo inclined) from whence they came, after they are once out of his poffeffion.

In this miftaken notion and ridiculous fyftem of breeding, fails every *penurious* and *mercenary* breeder, who, prompted by his own narrownefs of difpofition, affects to believe, there is little or no difference between *filling* and *feeding,* confidering a run *after the cows* as good as a *run with them*; that *chaff* is a much more *profitable* and healthy food than *oats*, and that an open farm-yard with a crib of barley or oat ſtraw, during the ſevere froſt and ſnow of a long dreary winter, are preferable to all other accommodations of food and ſhelter, as (to make uſe of his own juſtification) they are then in the moſt proper ſtate, " *a ſtate of nature*." Theſe are the *perſuaſive motives* aſſigned alſo by thoſe ſtrenuous advocates for general improvement, who barely ſubſiſt their mares during the tedious months of geſtation, under an idea perfectly coincident with the principles juſt deſcribed, that a mare after having been covered, requires but " *little or no keep*," as (with ſuch contemptible ſpeculators) the *act itſelf* is ridiculouſly ſuppoſed to make the mare *fat*. This is the invariable opinion among the leſs enlightened claſs of ruſtics ; and though the act and its conſequence may be juſtly ſaid to make the mare *big*, yet the original remark is certainly too ludicrous for ſerious conſideration.

After the neceſſary introduction of ſuch obſervations as are evidently connected with,

and

and branch directly from the subject, we return to the time best adapted by nature and the season to the foaling of the mare. A few words having been already interposed upon the inconvenience of dropping her foal *too early*, something consequently appertains to its falling *too late*; this should never happen when the year is too far advanced, as the *produce* then has to encounter hourly increasing difficulties, the daily declination of the genial sun, the decaying state of the verdure, the impending rains, bleak winds, long nights, foggy days, and the lank weak grass, form so strong a combination against improvement, (particularly if the winter should prove an additional stroke of severity) that the colt frequently feels the disadvantage, and constantly displays it by the deficiencies in frame and figure as before described.

Taking however the variation of different counties into the aggregate, to fix a criterion of time applicable to all parts, I should not hesitate a moment to pronounce the last week in April, and the three first in May, the most proper month in the year for mares to take the horse, provided it can be by any means

effected

effected ; to promote which, the following
methods fhould be adopted : It is generally
perceptible when a mare is *horfing*, and it is
likewife univerfally known fhe will then take
the horfe without farther trouble, *mutual confent* therefore renders animadverfion unneceffary ; but fhould the mare upon being brought
to the horfe, not make any *fhew*, on the contrary give proofs of denial by repeated kicking and other violent exertions, let her (after
fufficient *trials)* be taken away, and fome
addition be made to her keep ; give her a fubftantial feed of good oats and a pint of old
beans twice a day, continuing to offer her
the horfe once in three days till a compliance
is effected.

After which it will be neceffary to offer
her the horfe at the expiration of eight days
(that is, on the *ninth)* from the day of her
having been covered ; if fhe again take the
horfe (which is not at all uncommon) you
reckon from the laft time of covering, upon
a fuppofition no conception took place from
the firft copulation, and that it is confequently
obliterated. On the contrary, fhould fhe,
after *repeated offers,* perfevere in rejecting the
horfe,

horfe, the firft covering is then fuppofed to have been effectual; notwithftanding which, the mare, *in either cafe*, is to be produced and tried with the horfe at the end of a *fecond eight* days, when circumftances muft be regulated as at the end of the firft, entirely by her compliance or rejection.

Sentiments have varied exceedingly, upon the little probability of a mare conceiving when the act of copulation has been forcibly committed, without the leaft external difplay of defire, and in oppofition to the moft violent exertions of the mare. However my opinion might have originally fluctuated with the various reprefentations of others upon this fubject, I availed myfelf of an early opportunity to afcertain the fact, and remove any doubts that may have arifen within my own mind, although the recital will not perhaps render a repetition of the trial equally fuccefsful in the opinion of others; yet I have been fince repeatedly informed, the experiment is very frequently made, and not without its fhare of fuccefs.

In the year 1773, (refiding then at Hor-
E 3   fel,

fel, near Chobham, in Surrey,) ·I intended
covering two mares by *Woodcock*, half brother to Eclipse, that then remained at Eg-
ham, for the season; one of the mares took
the horse without reluctance, the other rejected him with the greatest violence; at the
expiration of time before mentioned, they
were again offered the horse and *both refused.* On the ninth day, I made the same
journey with the same success, and then concluded the mare that had been covered to be
perfectly safe; determined however, to make
no more journies of *uncertainty* upon the business, I asked TOWNSEND, the owner of
the horse, if he had any objection to let
the horse cover the mare compulsively, upon
condition she was so completely trammeled as
not to injure the horse? This being readily
agreed to on his part, and the mare *strongly
hobbled*, the horse was brought out, and being luckily very fresh, full of vigour, and eager as she was reluctant, the *leap* was obtained with much less difficulty than could
be possibly expected: At the end of the
eight days I again attended with the mare,
and found she rejected the horse with more
inveteracy than in any of my former journies.
I now

I now made up my mind to take no more trouble in the bufinefs, but leave the reft to chance ; in a very few months fhe was vifibly in foal, and produced me an exceeding handfome colt that I difpofed of at a high price to a gentleman in Norfolk, when rifing two years old.

This circumftance I have related, to eftablifh by proof the confiftency of adopting the *alternative*, when the feafon is fo far advanced as to hazard the lofs of the year by longer delay ; for my own part, (and it is clear I fpeak experimentally) I fhould never hefitate to cover a mare in this way, if fhe continued to refufe the horfe till the laft week in *May*, or the firft week in *June*, much rather chufing to *ravifh* the mafk of delicacy from her difpofition, than lofe her contribution to the ftock for that year, or have a colt fall fix weeks or two months too late in the feafon.

It will become perfectly applicable here, to introduce a few words refpecting the *exact period* of geftation in mares, upon which I never remember to have heard or read any thing

E 4

dicta-

dictatorially decisive more than the general affertion of their going *eleven months* (or the
common witticifm, that " a hare and a mare
go a *twelvemonth*") : But whether it is underftood eleven *lunar* or *calendar* months, I
believe has never been critically explained, (at
leaft generally known) and this is in fact the
more extraordinary when we recollect that
eleven calendar months make within two
days of *twelve* of the *other* ; nor indeed are
there but few inftances, in which the knowledge of fuch nice diftinction can be productive of much utility, yet it creates fome
furprife that it has not been particularly
noticed by fucceffive naturalifts, as circumftances have arifen and may fometimes happen, where fuch precifion would effectually
remove a doubt or eftablifh a fact.

A want of early attention to a difcovery of
this minutiæ was attended with a trifling lofs
to me fome years fince in my firft breeding
embarkation, when in poffeffion of much lefs
obfervation and experience ; for having obtained the loan of a ftrong boney mare from a
friend in Windfor Great Park, for the purpofe
of breeding, I had her covered by a large
powerful

powerful horfe then in the neighbourhood, and booked *the leap* according to cuftom; but having made no calculation of the calendar months, I kept her eleven lunar months and a fortnight (by the almanack) and not perceiving her to *fpring in the udder*, nor grow larger in the carcafe, I returned her (after taking the opinion of almoft every farmer and breeder in the country) upon a univerfal decifion, that, " fhe had no foal within her." The ultimate event proved *for once* the error of general judgment, for the owner (Mr. John-fon, then one of the keepers of the Great Park) taking a morning's walk among his ftock, found her with a fine colt foal at her foot in about ten days after her return, which proved a valuable horfe to him at five years old, that I had loft entirely by my inadver-tency and impatience.

The mare having taken the horfe but *once*, and that under my own eye (a truft I never delegated to another) added to the ftrict-eft attention in point of time, formed a com-bination to give proof, that a mare carries her young twelve *lunar* or eleven *calendar* months,

months, (which accurately taken are juſt the ſame) or that the exact given time varies in different ſubjects, and is ſo regulated by age or conſtitution, that there has yet been no criterion fixed for a nice diſtinction. The matter, however, if at all entitled to conſideration, may be moſt eaſily reduced to a certainty, by any gentleman having a variety of brood mares in his poſſeſſion, who will *note* thoſe that have taken the horſe but *once* in the ſeaſon, and take the trouble to book the day of their bringing forth; when by comparing *the whole*, the exact time of geſtation will be nearly demonſtrated, where no ſecond covering has intervened to render the deciſion imperfect.

The treatment of mares after being covered is regulated entirely by the claſs to which they belong; for having twice refuſed the horſe at the periods of time before ſtated, they are then ſaid to be *ſtinted*, and concluded in *foal*. But this is by no means always the caſe, for it frequently happens that ſuch mares produce no foals, although appearances are ſo much in their favour. *Thorough bred* mares (that is, mares whoſe blood is entirely untainted

tainted

tainted with any inferior crofs, and kept as
brood mares for the turf only) are thrown
out to grafs for the fummer feafon without
farther confideration; only taking particular
care that no geldings (or yearling colts) are
fuffered to accompany them in or near the
fame pafture, for fome few weeks after conception.

Mares of an inferior defcription in general ufe for the faddle, or thofe for agriculture, may be continued in their common employment with moderation, they feldom fuffer abortion but by great and improper exertions; they are therefore very frequently ufed
till within a few weeks of dropping their
burthen without the leaft fear of inconvenience. This is a fact fo univerfally eftablifhed,
that inftances have repeatedly happened of
mares obtaining *ftolen leaps* when out at pafture, without the knowledge and very much
againft the inclination of the owners; this
circumftance, from various motives, has been
confidered fo prejudicial, (where breeding has
not been intended) that different and powerful
methods have been adopted, as the adminiftration of *favine* in large quantities, violent exertions

ertions in drawing, or long and very fpeedy journies taken to promote abortion, and thofe without the leaft effect ; to corroborate which, the introduction of one only becomes at all necefſary, as it is too well authenticated to admit a doubt of its certainty.

Some few years fince Sulphur, a well known running horfe of the Duke of Cumberland's, having leaped the paddock pailing of an immenfe height in Windfor Park, covered a hunting mare of Mr. Jephs's (then refident at Sandpit Gate) in the fight of many labourers, who reported the occurrence. As hunting feafon approached fhe was perceptibly in foal ; this was what he by no means wifhed, and was fo much hurt at the awkwardnefs of the circumftance, that he continued to hunt her inceffantly, covering the *ftrongeft leaps* and taking the deepeft ground to obtain *abortion*.

The event however fufficiently proved the *folly* (not to add cruelty or prefumption) of oppofing nature in her niceft operations ; for all the feverity fo inconfiderately put in practice, never in the leaft hurt the mare, or debilitated

bilitated the fœtus: at her proper time fhe produced *a foal*, that (to render the circumftance more remarkable) at five years old won the *fifty pound plate* annually given for the keepers and yeoman prickers to be run for over Afcot.

This invincible ftamina or hardinefs of conftitution fo worthy recital in this inftance, is not (let it be underftood) fo entirely general as to be applicable to all the clafs without exception ; it therefore becomes perfectly in point to introduce a cafe in direct contraft, that may be likewife productive of utility, in preventing too great exertions with mares in fuch ftate, under a firm opinion that the lofs is lefs likely to happen than it really is and actually may.

Having about feven years fince purchafed of the breeder at *Horton* in *Buckinghamfhire*, a four year old mare got by *Bell's Denmark*, I obferved to him (during the negociation for purchafe) that from the depth of her carcafe and hollownefs of the flank, fhe was certainly early in foal ; on the contrary, he affured me, pofitively, no horfe had ever been near her,

her, and that it was merely the effect of laying at grafs. This mare, though fo young,
was a very excellent trotter; and having foon
after occafion to take a profeffional journey
with fome expedition, (the road being exceedingly good) I made obfervation by my watch
that fhe trotted the *feven miles* in five and
thirty minutes without the leaft *feeming* inconvenience; but on the morning following
I found fhe had *flipped* a colt foal very perfect of about three months conception, though
no extraordinary exertions were ufed on the
occafion.

The recital of cafes fo exactly in point lay
claim to the attention of breeders in general,
as they undoubtedly conftitute a bafis in experience, upon which the judgment may be
difcretionally formed at what time it will be
proper to difcontinue the working of fuch
mares, when it is clearly afcertained how
flight a portion of labour may endanger the
dam, and prove deftructive to the progeny.

The neceffary qualifications for procreation in both fire and dam having been fully in-
veftigated, and the blemifhes, defects, and local
contingencies, that tend to forbid the attempt
fairly

fairly explained, we come now to the crisis
of delivery, or the mare's bringing forth ; an
event so wonderfully accomplished by the almost unerring efforts of NATURE, that upon
the fairest calculation, not one mare in a
hundred suffers in any respect (more than the
temporary disquietude) from an exertion of
so much magnitude, although in the moments of reflection it absolutely becomes a
matter of admiration how the shock is sustained, without a much greater frequency of
the danger that so seldom ensues.

Notwithstanding this providential interposition for the safety of animals so little enabled to relieve themselves, it is worthy remark, that where difficulty and danger once
occur, the case becoming preternatural, it
generally terminates in the death of one or
the other, and not uncommonly in the destruction of both ; this may probably proceed from the construction of parts not being
generally understood, and the little chance
of assisting nature with the same ease and
accuracy as some other parts of the creation.

A loss of this description, after a year or
more

more of tedious hope and expectation, confequently produces temporary gloom and ferious difappointment; in fome inftances the dam becomes the victim, in others the foal; to the latter there is no palliative, to the former but one alternative: It is a cuftom almoft univerfal upon the death of the mare (foon after relief from her burthen) to defpair of fuccefs in raifing the foal by art, and it is frequently difpofed of without delay, that a circumftance fo unlucky may be the fooner erafed from memory and buried in oblivion.

This hafty decifion is by no means to be commended, although it is almoft generally known the power of inftinct is fo very predominant in this fpecies, that it muft be a fact exceedingly rare, to find a mare that will, by whatever ftratagem you can put in force, cherifh any other foal than her own; this moft undoubtedly arifes from their feldom or never producing a plurality of young at *one time*; a circumftance by no means uncommon with almoft every other animal of the creation, who are the more eafily impofed upon to nourifh and protect a fpurious offspring.

The

The general defpondency before-mentioned refpecting the furvivor, is not to be juftified where the foal is of value adequate to the trouble; nor indeed to be neglected upon the fcore of *humanity*, when unremitting induftry and perfeverance can fo readily furnifh an artificial fubftitute for maternal care and nutrition. It may be naturally concluded I allude to the great probability (and in fome cafes certainty) of bringing the foal up *by hand*; a remarkable inftance of which becomes immediately applicable, in the perfect recollection of a horfe bred by his late Royal Highnefs, William Duke of Cumberland, that at his death became the property of the celebrated Captain O'Kelly, and in the fucceffive poffeffion of both, for a feries of years, won more *give-and-take* plates than any other horfe in the kingdom.

The fact was exactly thus : The colt being the firft foal of a young mare that had been taken into the brood ftud without training, upon the produce of which his Royal Highnefs had formed great expectations, it proved matter of much furprife and difappointment (being totally repugnant to the reciprocal af-

fection in nature) that so soon as the colt
had fallen, the mare absolutely *took fright* at
her own offspring, and never could be once
brought to the least association with it whatever.   Every stratagem that could be devised
was put into practice under the immediate
inspection of his Royal Highness, to effect a
natural union between the dam and her foal,
but without the least probability of success ;
those fruitless efforts were therefore relinquished, and alternate attempts made to render the abandoned orphan a son of adoption
with different mares in rotation, but with no
prospect even of hope.   In this dilemma the
Duke, whose humanity in matters of much
greater importance will stand recorded to the
end of time, fully intent upon preserving the
colt if possible, (with a *declared* pre-senti-
ment of his future eminence) determined
upon his being brought up *by hand if possible*,
without a relative consideration to trouble or
expense, and issued his orders accordingly.
The event justified the endeavour, and the
success of the undertaking was transmitted
to posterity by the Royal Sponsor, with the
name of the horse ; for under the appellation
of MILKSOP, his very capital performances
                                    may

may be found in the " *Racing Calendar*," fo long as it fhall retain a place in the fporting libraries.

Circumftances of this kind happen, however, fo very rarely, that inftructions refpecting cafualties remote and unlikely, might be deemed fuperfluous, did not a vindication immediately arife from the exulting confolation, of knowing by what means to encounter fuch difficulties whenever they occur.

Returning therefore to the act of foaling, which, as before obferved, *generally happens* without the leaft danger or difficulty, and nine times out of ten in the night, it becomes the bufinefs of the owner or fuperintendant to difpofe the mare in fuch place of fafety, that mifchief is at leaft *not likely* to enfue; and this caution may prove the more acceptable, when it is recollected by every breeder, fportfman, or refident in the country, how very common it is in the feafon to hear of foals being *fmothered* in a ditch, or *drowned* in a rivulet, to the *poffibility of which*, the attention of the inadvertent owner had never been even

for

for a moment directed. It is likewise by no means inapplicable to obferve, that for fome days previous to the expected foaling of the mare, fhe fhould be kept in rather a fparing than plentiful fituation; to prevent a too great repletion of the inteftines and confequent compreffion upon the uterus, producing extreme pain, difficulty and delay in the delivery, which might otherwife never occur.

The mare having (as is generally the cafe) been freed from her burthen without inconvenience, and no circumftance arifing to forbid it, let her be immediately removed to a healthy and luxuriant pafture, calculated to furnifh not only a fufficiency of fupport for her own frame, but affording a fuperflux for the fubftantial and nutritious fupport of her young. In this a proper difcrimination is abfolutely neceffary; lank, fwampy, four grafs will certainly expand the frame, fubfift the dam, and contribute a flow of milk for the foal; but not of that rich and luxurious quality that is derived from feeding upon the fucculent herbage of maiden meadow, or upland grafs in high perfection;

fection ; both which contribute so very much to the daily growth and improvement of the colt, that it is a matter of the utmost consequence to the breeder, whose principal object should be to attain every possible advantage in *height*, *bone*, and *condition*, previous to the commencement of severe weather, during which growth is in general suspended, unless liberally promoted by the salutary interposition of good food, and proper shelter to encounter the inclemency of the season.

This is the first step to be taken where no disagreeable traits intervene to require a different mode of treatment ; but should the mare (by foaling before her time, or in severe sharp winds, a cold wet night, long and painful delivery, or other circumstances too abstruse to be discovered) visibly labour under *fixed dejection, bodily languor, loss of appetite,* laying down as if painfully weary, and totally inattentive to the infantile fondness of her foal ; it may be justly presumed, nature has sustained a severe shock from some one of the causes just recited, that cannot be too soon attended to and coun-

F 3   teracted,

teracted, for the prevention of more diftreffing confequences.

Fate is in general rapidly decifive in cafes
of this complexion, therefore delay (under
any pretence whatever) may prove not only
dangerous but deftructive ; the mare upon
fuch difcovery fhould be immediately removed, with her foal, to a ftill and com-
fortable fituation, as a large open ftable,
clofe cow-houfe, or bay of a barn, where
fhe fhould be expeditioufly fupplied with
fuch articles as invigorate the fyftem, encreafe the circulation, and recruit exhaufted
nature. About a gallon of water made warm
and impregnated with a portion of bran
or oatmeal, may be directly given to allay
the thirft which pain, fatigue, or difquietude never fails to excite, as well as to form
a kind of fubftitute during the preparation
of a plentiful mafh of malt, oats, and bran,
equal parts, into which fhould be ftirred
fix ounces of honey; this being given to the
mare, of confiftent warmth, will not only
gently ftimulate the debilitated powers
and gradually affift the ftrength, but promote an early flow of milk (for the gratification

fication of the expectant foal) which is always in some degree obstructed, if not totally suppressed, by the least indisposition of the dam.

The mash may be repeated twice every day, with plenty of the best hay, and occasional supplies of the water before-mentioned, till her recovery is sufficiently established, and the weather proportionably calm for her enlargement, in the way above-described, had no difficulty intervened. Should the same lassitude and dejection continue more than four and twenty hours after these methods have been adopted, bring into immediate use a dozen of the cordial pectoral balls from " The Gentleman's Stable Directory, Vol. I." and let one be given every night and morning in its prepared state, or dissolved in half a pint of gruel, and administered as a drink, or incorporated with each mash at the stated periods, till the whole are taken; continuing the aids of *mashes*, *warm water*, *nursing*, and *cloathing*, (if symptoms of great cold appear) till every appearance of complaint

plaint

plaint is removed, and nature perfectly re-
ftored.

Some mares, whether from a rigidity of the
veffels in not having their firft foals till an
advanced age, flight colds that obftruct the
fecretions, or whatever caufe unaffigned, are
very deficient in a neceffary flow of milk, by
which means the foal is deprived of perhaps
half the fuftenance requifite for his fupport
and expected improvement : This is a matter
well worthy minute infpection for the firft
three or four days after foaling, by which
time the food fhould be perfectly affimilated,
the lacteals expanded, and an ample fecretion furnifhed for the *full feed* of the foal.
This not being the cafe, fuch deficiency
fhould be very early difcovered, and as
eagerly affifted when known,

The richeft and moft luxuriant pafture
that can be obtained, with good foft
water at will, is the firft and beft natural ftep to remove fuch obftruction in its
infancy ; *that*, upon obfervation, not fucceeding in the defired degree, and the
colt

colt becoming perceptibly *ſtinted,* (which
may be plainly perceived not only by his
external appearance, but inceſſant attempts
to obtain ſupplies without ſuccefs) artificial
means muſt be adopted to ſolicit a due diſcharge of this very neceſſary fluid, without
which every expectation of the foal's growth
and gradual improvement muſt be rendered
abortive.

This object can only be accompliſhed by
enlarging the mode and encreaſing the means
of conveying a larger portion of more nutritious aliment into the ſyſtem ; from the general diffuſion of which, the lymphatics and
lacteals become proportionally diſtended, and
are conſequently enabled to ſecrete and diſcharge a much greater quantity than nature
in her more reluctant ſtate ſeems inclined to
beſtow.

This ſyſtematic procefs of nature may, to
the lefs enlightened reader, ſeem matter of
ſo much ambiguity, that ſomewhat more in
explanation may be probably required ; but
as abſtruſe reaſoning and phyſical definition
(it has been before ſaid) is not the purpoſe
of

of the prefent publication, every irrelative matter will be carefully avoided that can tend to perplex the mind or embarrafs the judgment. It would, therefore, be deviating widely from the plan originally formed for the accommodation of general comprehen-fion, were we (by unneceffary introduction) to enter into the very extenfive field of ana-tomical ftructure and animal mechanifm, demonftrating phyfically by what admirable means the excrementitious part of aliment is rejected from the ftomach and conveyed through the inteftinal canal, when divefted of its more fubtle and nutritious properties ; which being totally abforbed by an infinity of veffels in the very work of digeftion, is carried into the circulation, and there confti-tutes, by its different fecretions, the fource of life and fupport ; from which fyftematic transformation is derived that formation of blood, that gradual enlargement of flefh and bone, only to be explained by much literary information on one fide, and underftood by no fmall portion of medical knowledge on the other.

It will confequently fuffice to fay, that the

the reader, whose mind is more enlarged, whose views are more extensive, and who cannot reconcile his opinion or found his judgment upon the quality of *aliment*, the procefs of *digeftion*, or the effect of *nutrition*, by what has been concifely introduced upon thofe fubjects, muft derive more fubftantial affiftance from the variety of excellent profeffional publications more particularly adapted to fuch inveftigation and enquiry; as the majority of thofe who do me the honour of occafional infpection, will certainly expect, under the head we now write upon, to find much more matter of amufement and rural inftruction than fcientific difquifition.

Declining, therefore, a matter of fo much extent, and fo little applicable to the prefent purpofe, we naturally revert to the ftate of the mare and the means of enlarging the powers; from which alone, the foal is to receive not only a fufficiency of nutriment for bare fubfiftence, but an abfolute abundance or fuperflux for the promotion of advantages we have fo particularly explained. The deficiency before-mentioned having been attentively

attentively afcertained, and excellent pafture with good water not being found to
increafe the flow of milk fo much as is
evidently required, an addition of more fubftantial and nutritive food muft be affociated
with what has been always confidered the
firft and moft natural aliment for equeftrian
improvement.

All rules, however eftablifhed, are perpetually liable to fome exception, and nature is
not uncommonly affifted (or counteracted)
by ways and means the very leaft expected ;
for every conftitution will not be acted upon
in the fame manner either in the human or
brute creation. In fact, daily experience
with the human fpecies affords ample proof,
that the *fame articles* in phyfic or food fhall
act in a direct contrary way, and produce
a very different effect upon one habit to
what it fhall in another : A circumftance fo
generally known and admitted, would furnifh fufficient latitude for conjecture refpecting the animal we now treat of, was
proof really wanting to eftablifh fuch
opinion, which is by no means the cafe,
as numerous inftances might be quoted to
corroborate

corroborate a variety of similar contrasts, were they at all neceffary, to confirm a belief of what in reality there cannot be the leaft doubt of.

Convinced, therefore, of fuch facts, it is but a natural inference to conclude, the beft, or indeed pafture of any kind may not be fo equally conducive to the improvement and condition of *all immediately after foaling*, but that it may act as a powerful reftorative upon one, while it relaxes and debilitates the fyftem of another; particularly where, from a vitiated or difeafed ftate of the ftomach and inteftines, it paffes fo rapidly and indigefted through the body, as to depofit but little of either *effence* or *fubftance* for the fubfiftence of the frame or fupport of the foal.

This is undoubtedly one of the predominant caufes of the defect, and fhould be counteracted by fuch means as are calculated to ftrengthen the digeftive powers, animate the circulation, and diffufe a plentiful fupply of chyle to preferve the neceffary fecretions, without which a healthy and improving

proving ftate is not to be expected. To effect this, give a warm mafh every morning compofed of brown malt three quarts, and one of cracked oatmeal, (commonly called grits) let the water be poured on boiling hot, and repeatedly ftirred up till of a proper warmth, when it may be given in either field or ftable, unlefs any feverity of weather fhould render the latter moft eligible. In the evening of each day, give half a gallon of good found mealy oats, with the addition of a pint of old beans, either whole or fplit, as will be moft readily taken by the fubject for whom they are intended; thefe feeds, exclufive of their great nutritive property, will powerfully affift in retaining the aliment in the ftomach by their reftringent quality, thereby contributing largely to the general purport of the whole.

This plan fhould be perfevered in for fix days without intermiffion, when an increafed fupply of milk from the mare may be earneftly expected; but fhould that improvement not become perceptible, fhe may be reafonably deemed *a very poor nurfe*, and no other extraordinary means be attempted to affift the

the imperfection; but care muft be taken to wean the foal very early in the enfuing winter, (as will be hereafter explained) upon a well juftified prefumption, that at the autumnal declination of grafs, her flender portion of fupport for the foal will difappear alfo.

How far it may be confiftent, at leaft prudent, to breed *a fecond time* from mares whofe powers are evidently deficient in furnifhing fuch portion of milk as is abfolutely neceffary to ftamp the attempt with fuccefs, muft be left entirely to the decifion of the parties interefted in the event; fome of whom I have before obferved, are, from different motives, too much attached to undeferving favourites ever to fuffer their opinions to be warped by any confideration or remonftrance whatever. For my own part, I feel juftified by perfonal experience and attentive obfervation, in again making public declaration, that in fo ferious and expenfive a bufinefs as breeding for either the turf, field, road, or draft, no blind prejudice or infatuating prepoffeffion fhould influence me to perfevere in the practice with palpable points, defects, or difqualifications

against

under the disadvantage of bleak winds and frigid showers, but before there is a single blade of exuberant pasture to subsist the dam, or encourage the growth of twelve months tedious expectation.

From what has been so lately and repeatedly urged respecting the properties of different kinds of aliment, and its effect upon the animal system, little more can be required to prove, that whenever a necessity absolutely exists for subsisting the mare entirely upon *dry food*, the secretion of milk must be inevitably reduced, and the improvement of the foal proportionally obstructed. Taking this then as a matter universally admitted, and, in fact, what no man living will attempt to disprove, we may naturally conclude no rational investigator of truth and consistency will ever deviate so much from the line of his own interest, as to promote the propagation of what must, at the time of its birth, be in a great degree deprived of its most natural means of existence; a deficiency not in his power to supply by any adequate substitute whatever.

Relin-

Relinquifhing therefore fo extravagant an idea, we proceed to the time moft natural for bringing the mare to the horfe after her foaling, if fhe is intended to continue her fervices as a brood mare, and to be managed accordingly. The time moft applicable in one refpect, may not prove always the moft convenient in another, as it fhould be regulated, if poffible, to avoid the before mentioned extremes of the foal falling too early or late in the feafon. Moft mares will take the horfe on either the *ninth*, *fifteenth*, *twenty-firft*, or *twenty-feventh* day after foaling; of thefe, neither will occafion any great variation in the time of her foaling the next feafon; though I fhould adhere to either of the *two laft*, unlefs the mare had foaled late in the year, when the *firft* or *fecond* fhould certainly be preferred. After which covering, or refufal of the horfe, fhe fhould continue to be tried at the ftated periods fo particularly fpecified in the earlier part of the work; always concluding the mare to be ftinted, and in a ftate of conception, when fhe has repeatedly declined the horfe in the manner there defcribed.

G 2

Before

Before we take leave of this part of our
fubject, it comes directly in point to offer
a few words upon the almoft univerfal
practice of continuing to breed year after
year, from the fame mare, till nature over-
driven thwarts the attempt by the occafional introduction of a barren year, in direct
oppofition to the intent of the breeder, demonftrating upon *compulfion* the neceffity of
what he did not intend to comprehend by
choice.

The very means by which the embryo is
generated, and the nutriment required, not
only to fupport its growth during the
months of geftation, but the fubfequent
term of its *fuction*, evidently point out the
confiftency of fome portion of reft or re-
fpite for the dam, to acquire additional
ftrength, after the inceffant labour of continually collecting a double portion of food
to fubfift herfelf and fupport her off-
fpring.

The fafhionable and predominant plea of
attachment to intereft and felf-prefervation,
will render deaf to this remonftrance numbers

bers, who, unwilling to "lose the year," and incapable of imbibing inſtruction from the niceſt laws of nature, will be regulated implicitly by the dictates of their own mercenary ſenſations; affecting to believe, that the mare producing *a foal every year,* will continue her ſtock equally ſtrong, healthy, and valuable, with thoſe that are favoured with occaſional and neceſſary in-termiſſions. This is not the fact; attentive obſervation, accurate eſtimate, and impartial deciſion, will clearly prove ſuch ſucceſſion to degenerate in bone, ſize, ſtrength, and value, when produced from the ſame mare for a ſeries of years without the leaſt ceſſation; while, on the contrary, *a ſingle year's fallow* in every three or four, will, upon compariſon critically made, prove in the aggregate decidedly in favour of the breeder.

Having gone regularly through every branch of information at all appertaining to the propagation and preſervation of ſtock, we now come to the time and man-ner of *weaning;* a matter that muſt ever be regulated much more by the circumſtances of of the cafe than the ftate of the feafon, depending in a great degree upon the conditions we proceed to explain. Confiderations upon this fubject are fo unavoidably complex, and depend fo much upon contingencies, that a nicety of difcrimination is upon all occafions neceffary how to proceed in the bufinefs before us.

The difference of a mare foaling early or late in the feafon; her remaining fallow, or having taken the horfe and renewed her conception; the forward growth and rapid improvement, or puny and backward ftate of the foal, are all *conditional matters* upon which variations are to be formed. For inftance, where the mare has dropped her foal early in the feafon, has again taken the horfe, and the foal at her foot has improved properly, and acquired the defired ftrength and fize previous to the commencement of fevere weather; fuch foal fhould be taken from the dam fo foon as the decay of pafture perceptibly occafions a reduction in the fupply of milk; and this feparation becomes the more immediately neceffary upon an eftablifhed truth, that the
longer

longer a foal is permitted to oppress nature, by a compulsive secretion and evacuation of milk from a mare again advanced in foal, the more will the subject *in embryo* be consequently impoverished and restrained, when deprived of its portion of nutriment, *then* converted through another channel, and appropriated to a different use. This incontrovertible system of the animal œconomy must be so evidently clear to the most uncultivated comprehension, (accustomed to dedicate but little attention to the slightest indications of nature) that it becomes matter of admiration how so absurd a practice can ever be supported upon the basis of inadvertency; when it would be rendering nature accessary to a perversion of her own laws, even to suppose it was ever intended, that any animal existing should longer subsist or *prey* upon the *very vitals* of its dam, when the frame was again advancing in pregnancy with another.

From this necessary allusion to a practice that is not only exceedingly common and too little attended to, but is also prejudicial to the subjects themselves in a greater

G 4

degree

degree than generally underftood, (merely for want of a little fcientific reflection upon the properties of food and its different effects) we come to a cafe appofite in itfelf, that muft be regulated accordingly; as, where the mare has foaled late in the year, and has not been again put to horfe, or where the retarded and unpromifing ftate of the foal renders extra care and nurfing abfolutely neceffary : In either of which, every encouragement fhould be given to promote the ftrength and growth of the foal, during the inclemency of the winter feafon, which, it fhould be remembered, he is not nearly fo well enabled to encounter, as thofe of a greater age poffeffing the advantages before defcribed. In fuch inftances as thefe, although the flow of milk from the dam will be very confiderably checked by the alteration of food dependent upon the different feafons, yet with frequent fupplies of good hay to the mare, it may be proportionally affifted, and with occafional aids of proper food to the foal, great advantages may be derived from letting them run together through the feverer months of the winter; to evade the ill effects

effects of which, nocturnal shelter will very much contribute.

Notwithstanding every possible information that can be introduced, such variety of cases may occur with so great a complication of circumstances, that no literary description, however diffuse, can prove completely adequate to every idea upon the subject; conditional instructions must always become subservient to the discriminating judgment of the owner or superintendant, upon whose favourable opinion or prejudice, *caprice* or *compliance*, will depend the effect of the whole; and to such precarious decision alone, must the writer ultimately submit the consistency and execution of his directions, though he were to produce an *immaculate volume* upon the subject.

Conscious however of the compulsive necessity for such dependence, and the diversity of cases requiring conditional changes to the variety of circumstances that may occur, no particular *week* or *month* can be invariably fixed for weaning; as some of the contingencies before-mentioned may render it unavoid-

unavoidably neceffary in the earlieft month
of the winter, or protract it to the lateft in
the fpring; which muft, after all that can
be offered in print, depend entirely upon
the difcretion and intereft of the parties
more immediately concerned.

Waving, for thofe reafons, farther animadverfion refpecting the *time*, we advert
to the *manner* of effecting a change fometimes attended with difficulty, but feldom or
never with danger, particularly when regulated by due attention to *circumftances, feafon, ftate,* and *condition;* confiderations that
never efcape the eye of vigilance, and generally infure their own reward. Towards
the conclufion of the year, the foal acquires,
by inftinct and obfervation, fome relifh for
pafture, but unluckily begins to enjoy it
juft at its autumnal declination, when long
dreary nights, damp fogs, and frequent
rains have fucceeded the enlivening rays
of the genial fun, depriving it of its former fubftance and vernal fweetnefs; at
this critical period all nature undergoes a
vifible alteration, and the change is as fe-

vere

vere in its effects upon the animal as the vegetative part of the world.

In this general revolution, the expected and former nutriment from the *dam* becomes not only reduced in *quantity*, but impaired in *quality*; divested in a great degree of its balsamic and nourishing property, it wisely points out to the foal, the *feeling* necessity of an adequate substitute for such deficiency; under so predominant a sensation as *hunger*, he readily submits to an alteration in the means of subsistence, and in a few days becomes perfectly reconciled to the food allotted him, provided it is applicable to the state of his infancy, good in its kind, and properly selected to gratify the calls of nature.

Of these there are various kinds, that have each their different advocates, whether in *oats, bran, chaff, barley, wheat, hay,* or *straw,* and each advocate loaded with reasons of the first importance and self consequence, (regulated perhaps by pecuniary sensation) to justify the opinion he has formed: But as it is by no means the purpose

pose to lead our readers through a dull and tedious labyrinth of perplexities, without a glimmering of either *utility* or *information*, we shall endeavour to ascertain the preference without animadverting upon the judgment and opinion of others, wishing upon the basis of truth and consistency *only* to establish the criterion of our own.

It has been generally said of OATS (although the universally established food for horses) that they are dangerous to foals at the time of weaning, under an idea of the *optic nerves* being so violently affected by the strength required in mastication, as to occasion future disease, debilitation, and sometimes loss of the eyes: As this is however a matter that can never be reduced to certainty, but must always remain dependent upon conjecture, without even the possibility of proof, it may be perfectly applicable to the disposition of those who entertain doubts, to adopt the alternative of feeding with the *grain* or *grits* only first divested of the hulls, as in the *shell* or *husk* such difficulty must be resident, and not in the meal.

BRAN

BRAN may have its occasional use, when called in aid of other *aliment*, but is entitled to little or no estimation on the score of *nutriment*, being like the different kinds of *straw* or *chaff*, evidently calculated more to amuse the appetite and expand the frame than subsist the body. BARLEY, (particularly when manufactured, and meliorated into malt) as well as WHEAT, commands the priority of invigoration with almost every part of the creation; for whether the experiment be made on *man, beast*, or the more inferior classes of *fowl*, or *vermin*, it becomes every way conspicuous. The great salubrity and nutritive property of sound, fragrant, well-made MEADOW and CLOVER HAY are too universally known to require a single line upon their excellence.

In addition to these, most of which are in constant use, may be introduced two articles equally applicable, though not in such general request; they are nevertheless in the highest estimation with those who have proved their utility, and stand entitled to the warmest recommendation, First, the *pulse* passing under the denomination of
HORSE

HORSE BEANS, which from their great
fubftance, adhefive quality, and known invigorating power, are juftly fuppofed to
convey a greater portion of nutriment to
the fyftem than any other corn appropriated to the fame ufe. Admitting this to
be really the cafe, they likewife retain the
advantage of being readily adapted to horfes
of every defcription from infancy to age,
and may be given as exigencies require, either in their natural ftate whole, or *fplit*, as
is the ufual method when given with bran (a
feed very common with horfes of the lower
clafs of mechanics) or completely ground,
(and called *bean meal*) for the ufe of foals or
colts, fo young that they are incapable of
receiving them in any other ftate.

The other article, whether recommended
as a ufeful winter fubftitute for the more
fucculent herbage of the fummer, or only
as a cheap and additional method of fubfiftence, need only be more generally known
to eftablifh its own reputation; whether
joined to the accuftomed food of draft
horfes ufed in agriculture, colts during
thofe months of the year when the growth
of

of pasture is restrained, foals when weaning, or in addition to the keep of mares whose foals are required and permitted to run at the foot *all the winter*, it is of equal utility, particularly to the latter, whose flow of milk it greatly enlarges if given in sufficient quantities to promote the advantage.

CARROTS, the article thus highly commended, after fair and impartial trial, is one of the most valuable in the vegetable world, and so easy of cultivation, that in a light sandy soil no crop is supposed to produce a greater share of emolument; of this, certain adventurers are so well convinced, that the very labourers in the north-west parts of the county of Surry, rent from the neighbouring farmers a moiety of even the poorest land upon the verge of the barren heath, at the exorbitant price of three and four pounds per acre for the summer season, only to produce a single crop, when it is immediately resigned to the landlord for his season of wheat to follow.

The

The largest and handsomest they begin to pull in September and October; these are very neatly formed into bunches, and consigned to the London market by the waggon load, at the enormous expence of *two guineas* for the carriage only, which with the additional trouble and charge of double *hoeing, pulling, washing,* and *bunching,* gives it the appearance of a very expensive crop; but when it is taken into the calculation, that *three,* sometimes *four* loads are produced from a single acre, that (according to the season) sell in London, from *four* to *six* pounds per load, the great advantage becomes palpably striking even to the most indifferent arithmetician. But the emolument ends not here; for upon the average, no more than two-thirds of the produce are included in the above proportion, as turning out sufficiently handsome for the trade before described; the remaining proportion, that are *short, ill-shaped* and *forked,* are deemed *refuse,* and used in the winter by such growers as have stock of their own, or disposed of by those who have none to their neighbours at a very moderate price. To the corroboration of

this

this fact I speak experimentally, having been a consumer among my own stock of *four-score bushels* in one winter, purchased at only sixpence each bushel, exclusive of a very considerable quantity produced from a part of my own land, then under similar cultivation from a thorough conviction of their utility and profit.

The method to preserve them for the winter consumption is as follows: Let them be taken up early in the autumn, so soon as their superficial or vegetative parts begin to decline, and laid upon a bed of *new wheat straw,* (in a dry room or close granary) without cleaning, just as they are taken out of the ground; they are then to be plentifully covered with the same bedding, to protect them from long and severe frosts that frequently ensue, after being affected by which, they soon decay and become rotten; no fear of this need, nevertheless, be entertained, provided proper care and attention be paid to the bed and covering, as they then continue perfectly found to the expiration of a very long winter. There is also another equally effectual method of prefervation much in ufe in the neighbourhood alluded to, by fub-ftituting *fand* for ftraw, letting them be very fubftantially covered to exclude the external air; but as that article is not fo univerfal, or to be obtained by any means in many parts of the kingdom, ftraw muft undoubtedly prove moft convenient for the purpofe.

During the feafon required for confump-tion, let any quantity be taken from the heap and placed in a mafh or other tub, there covered with water from a pump, or pond, as may be moft convenient; when having ftood an hour or two, to foften the furrounding earth left on for prefervation, they fhould be well wafhed with a heath broom for a few minutes, till properly clean; then pouring off the foul water, and wafh-ing them once more with a pail or two of clean, they will foon become dry enough for the following operation.

Let them be cut firft longitudinally, then tranfverfely; or, to make ufe of a more comprehenfible term, (at leaft rather better

adapted

adapted to the ruftic capacities of thofe likely to become the operators) " *athwart and acrofs*," into fmall fquares about the fize of a horfe or tick bean; in which ftate they will be confumed in the winter with the greateft avidity, by any clafs of horfes, mares, or colts, either alone or intermixed with chaff, oats, bran, or any other dry food to which they are accuftomed.

To remove fuch doubts as may arife in the minds of thofe who pafs through life in the true *mechanical dog-trot* of their great grandfires, and who, from their perfonal pride and innate dulnefs, never condefcend to make an *experiment*, or fanction an *improvement* when made; I think it neceffary to repeat the fact, that I have with the greateft fuccefs introduced this additional article of food to all the different horfes in my poffeffion (hunters excepted) during a long, dreary, and fevere winter, never remembering to have had them in better health, vigour, and condition. Among thefe were a team of draft horfes in conftant employment, not only in agriculture but occafional hard work upon

H 2   , the

the road; growing colts of different kinds, as well as brood mares and foals, who all equally enjoyed a participation of the experiment in every kind of way it could be offered them; tending fufficiently to juftify every thing I can prefume to offer in recommendaion of the practice, more particularly with ftock required only in *improving condition* during the winter, and not deftined to any kind of labour.

In this juft reprefentation, I beg by no means to have my expreffions mifconftrued or my meaning perverted, but defire it fhould be generally underftood, I urge their utility in applicable proportions as a cheap auxiliary to *other food*, without indulging an idea of their being ufed *alone*; as well as to have it held in remembrance, however ferviceable and healthy they may have proved, and certainly are to the unemployed part of ftock, it was never my intent to declare them capable of conftituting *the bafis of nutrition and fupport* for horfes in conftant and laborious work. On the contrary, knowing experimentally the great expence of breeding, and how neceffary it

is

is to acquire occasional aid from the frequent interpofition of *æconomy*, I earneftly recommend the culture of them upon that fcore, (in thofe parts of the kingdom not fo favourably adapted to breeding) as a very ufeful and profitable affociate with other food for brood mares, foals, and growing colts, in fevere or long winters, when hay and corn are at an exceeding high price from a general failure in the crop, or an indifferent feafon for the harveft.

From this unavoidable deviation we return to the bufinefs of WEANING, a matter that will be in fome degree more eafily reconciled by permitting the foal to feed with the mare for a few days upon the dry food previous to the entire feparation. The queftion naturally and indeed generally arifing at this period, is not, what food is the moft falutary for the fubject in queftion; but, Which is the kind of food moft applicable to the fenfations of the owner? Though was reafon or prudence confulted, that food would be adopted moft adequate to the probable value of the foal; for notwithftanding all that can be urged in the defence of breeding

H 3   fyftem-

fyftematically, to produce ftock of fhape,
ftrength, figure, fafhion, bone or fpeed (according to the purpofes for which they are
defigned) there will ftill remain a more than
moderate proportion of the breeders formerly
defcribed, who muft inevitably continue to propagate ftock, not worth the *proper fupport* of
even the firft twelve months, was their intrin-
fic value to be brought into arbitrative competition with the year's confumption.

No doubt can be entertained but the fweet-
eft hay, with a daily portion of the hulled
oats and a trifling addition of the bean meal,
would be as perfectly grateful to the weaning foal of a *five pound pony mare* as to the
palate of a fon of HIGHFLYER; but it is
natural to conclude, in the prefent hourly
increafing age of fagacity and penetration,
felf-intereft, with its concomitants, will never
be fo totally obfcured, as not to regulate the
conduct of the majority, and that mares and
colts will in general be fupported with a
political reference to *profit* and *lofs*, however
fome exceptions (with favourites of a former
defcription) may produce many a four-year
old at the domeftic expence of *thirty*, *forty*

or

or *fifty pounds*, whofe whole accumulation of *points* and *perfections* will never exceed *five and twenty* when brought to the teft of infpection at a public market.

Confcious how many will continue to breed under every difadvantage, and to perfift under every peculiarity, I fhall fubmit the diftinct kind of aliment to be felected, and the quantity to be regulated entirely by the judgment, whim, caprice, experiment, or local cuftom of every individual, upon a perfect conviction he will juftly claim and exert that privilege, in oppofition to any opinion or dictation of mine; whofe farther inftructions upon this head might be candidly confidered obtrufive, where conditional directions under fo many contingencies (as the ftate of various fubjects and temperature or feverity of different feafons) muft prove totally inadequate to general application.

Convinced however, on the contrary, how very many there are, who anxious for information and open to inftruction, poffefs patience to receive, and judgment to adopt, every fpecies of improvement calculated for the promotion

H 4

of

of general good; it is intirely for their accommodation, that I have minutely defcended not only to an explanation of the quality of different kinds of food, but repeatedly to the work of digeftion and effect of nutrition, that the very means of *growth, ftrength* and *condition* may be more rationally confidered and fundamentally underftood.

Prefuming on the care taken to inculcate fuch knowledge, and thoroughly convinced of the advantages that arife from a liberal diftribution of provender to ftock of every kind upon certain emergencies, I beg to conclude my obfervations under this head, with an additional injunction to breeders of every denomination, to endeavour in the *two firft winters,* to acquire all poffible advantage in fize, ftrength, and bone; which I have before faid, and again affert, depends as much upon the judicious and plentiful fupplies of food, as the qualifications of horfe or mare, fo folely relied upon and eternally echoed by thofe fubordinate cavilifts who poffefs the opinion, but not the means, to juftify their affertion. For fize, ftrength and bone being thus conftantly promoted by care and attention,

tion, they not only form the frame for a ready acquifition of flesh in that feason of the year when nature difpenfes her gifts with a more liberal hand, but being *once obtained* can never be obliterated; while, on the contrary, the first opportunity of acquiring thofe perfections being totally loft by an unfair reftraint in fuftenance during the *firft two years*, the ftock is more or lefs *ftinted*, and an irreparable deficiency conftituted that can never be fupplied in *the fame fubjects*, by either prefent regret or future repentance.

BREAKING.

IT will not come within the limits of this work, or the intention of the writer, to interfere with the operative part of the art, offering a differtation upon the routine of *leading, lunging, backing, riding, mounting,* or *difmounting,* with *eafe, grace,* and *agility;* thefe are the profeffional privileges of BREAKERS alone, from the ruftic rough rider of the moft obfcure village in the country, to the fafhionable and accomplifhed MENAGE MASTER GENERAL of the metropolis.

tropolis. Proffefing therefore no interference
with, or attack upon, the principles of the
fcience, I proceed to fuch allufive remarks
and inferences as intereft not only breeders and
fportfmen, but all thofe who have any immediate intercourfe with the fpecies, whether
from the motive of attachment, pleafure,
health, or bufinefs.

The firft object for general confideration,
is the age moft proper for bringing into work
horfes of different defcriptions, according to
their diftinct appropriations; but this, like
moft other matters, has become fubfervient
to the prevalence of fafhion, and in much
lefs than half a century undergone a total
revolution. Some years fince (and not a
great many) colts and fillies were haltered
and handled a little *at three*; turned out
again and completely broke *at four*; ufed moderately during their *fifth year*, and thought
to be fufficiently matured for conftant work *at
fix*; fuch fyftem has been, however, gradually changing as the value of horfes continued to increafe, a circumftance that in all
probability effected the alteration, by tempt-
ing breeders to turn their ftock into fpecie,
with much lefs trouble, expence and anxiety
than

than when kept fo long upon hand before they could be taken to market.

This has turned fo much to advantage in their annual transfer to the London dealers, who purchafe at the famous fairs of Banbury, Northampton, Leicefter, Reading, and many others, (exclufive of their extenfive agencies in Yorkfhire and other diftant counties) that they are now broke and fold fo foon as they have obtained *fize,* and undergo the moft infamous practices upon their teeth, to enable the *confcientious feller* to difpofe of a two, three, or four year old, for a *four, five,* or *fix*; which he frequently does with fuch affurances of *truth* and *integrity,* that the cheat is very little likely to be difcovered by any fagacity or circumfpection whatever.

A fimilar degree of refinement has been effected upon the turf, as with the more inferior claffes; for what has been promoted by *intereft* on one hand, has been extended by the invincible *fpirit of oppofition* on the other. It is but few years fince a four year old plate was confidered the firft *public* trial of fpeed and bottom, between young horfes

calculated

calculated and trained for racing: But horfes (as well as women) are, by the great and il-lumined effect of modern penetration, found to be fo much forwarder in the *natural ftate* of their conftitution, that they are brought into ufe many years fooner in the present than the paft century; having now not only plates conftantly run for by three years old, but frequent matches and fweepftakes with two years old and yearlings.

In this general improvement (if it can be fo termed) I believe any obfervant or experi-enced reader will coincide with me in opinion, and hazard the affertion, that many hundred horfes are annually crippled or irrecoverably injured before they arrive at maturity; that is, before they arrive at a proper age for the work to which they are fo frequently moft injudicioufly deftined. In fupport of this fact, no greater or more indifputable au-thority need be adduced, than a reference to the infinity of invalids to be daily feen on all the popular roads leading to the metropolis; but fhould a ftronger proof be required, to meet the opinions of the *interefted* and *incre-dulous*, let it be extracted from the vifible effect

effect of the burning cautery, or rotational multiplicity of FIRED HORSES in perpetual liberation from the hands of every eminent operator in the various parts of the kingdom. As this custom is now too far advanced in practice, and too firmly established by interest, (at the original source of circulation) to admit of cure or palliation, farther animadversion upon its ill effects cannot be productive of either success or utility; continuing therefore our determination to avoid remarks extraneous or desultory, we proceed to such practical observations as are more likely to excite general attention.

Of these, none become more entitled to the consideration of *horse breakers* and their employers, than the natural disposition and temper of the subject they are taking in hand; for it is a positive fact that more horses have been injured in their tempers and dispositions by the indiscretion, impetuosity, or *professional intoxication* of those to whose management they are unavoidably entrusted, than by any other means whatever.

Reason and observation afford evident demonstration

monstration that horses have their different degrees of sagacity and penetration; their spontaneous efforts are all regulated by the most impressive and inherent sensations, dependent upon passions conspicuous as our own; subject to an equal display of fortitude, fear, joy, grief, courage, timidity, attachment and prejudice as any of the human species; and this is so perfectly known to those who have made nature the object of frequent meditation, that they cannot consider the communication a matter of novelty; while those who receive the information under an impression of doubt, must, in the moments of reflection, be seriously convinced they have read but little in the fertile volume of experience.

Upon the most palpable conviction, that those passions have a predominant ascendancy over their different subjects, I presume to urge the consistency of rendering the animal obedient to the will, by such methods as are calculated more to acquire his submission than excite his anger; or, in other words, to accomplish the business more by gentle means than coercive exertions. The necessity fity for earneftly recommending this lenity in the practice, has arifen from innumerable inftances within my own knowledge, of horfes rendered invincibly reftiff by the dint of perpetual ill ufage and unjuft oppofition; when from the natural bent of their difpofitions, a different mode of treatment would have produced a direct contrary effect.

To this part of the fubject I have ever paid the greateft perfonal attention, and declare, with the ftricteft adherence to truth, I never yet faw a *reftiff horfe* made better by violence and abufe. If any vociferous difputant, fond of difplaying his courage and exerting his power, feels his *innate cruelty* in fome degree abridged by the intervention of humanity, and arrogantly afks, "Whether he is to abandon his purpofe, and permit the horfe to gain the victory and become his mafter?" I anfwer him with the greateft ferenity, "On no account whatever." Such is not the purport of my recommendation; our intents are undoubtedly the fame, but to be eventually accomplifhed by very different means; I repeatedly urge the propriety of due attention to the various tempers and difpofitions positions of horses, upon the purest conviction, that the treatment really necessary for a horse of very high courage and almost invincible spirit, cannot be confistent or proper for one of extreme timidity; that one horse may be subdued from any 'predominant vice, or regulated to any particular action, by a moderate exertion of power, while another will submit only to a constant display of the greatest tenderness and familiarity. These extremes frequently exist in horses of a similar class, value, speed, and qualifications; equally liable to injurious impressions from being managed in a way directly opposite to the very nature of their dispositions.

A due degree of patient discrimination should be always exerted, to discover the temper of the subject and ascertain the line of distinction; what may be expected from a steady firmness and persuasive mildness, previous to the too ready exertion of *violence*, in general very eagerly conceived and maliciously executed. Horses are perfectly conscious of the different treatment they receive, and give the most striking proofs of their attachment or dislike in consequence:

This

This is a fact but little known amidst the multitude of *superficial observers* and *metropolitan sportsmen*, but incontrovertible with those who survey this animal with the daily eye of exquisite pleasure and admiration.

The *equanimity, fortitude,* and *sobriety,* so indispensibly necessary for the successful breaking and management of young, restiff, timid, or high spirited and refractory horses, must be too sensibly felt by every judicious Reader, to require the least animadversion upon the advantage of such qualifications; I shall therefore proceed to a few remarks upon the almost systematic conduct of grooms, breakers, and servants, (to whose care horses of the first estimation are unavoidably entrusted) who persisting indiscriminately to effect all their purposes *by force,* frequently err much more from the very motive that Pope's rustic hero whistled, " *want of thought,* " than any pre-determined spirit of opposition to the rules of consistency and discretion.

It is no uncommon occurrence with constant travellers, to perceive one of this description mounted upon a horse denominated

reftiff, that without any apparent motive (at leaft perceptible to the rider) by which the caufe may be difcovered, fuddenly *ftop, retreat,* or *turn round* upon the road, vifibly encreafing his reluctance to go forward, in proportion to the anger and violent oppofition of the rider ; who, too frequently a flave to irafcibility, rafhly fuppofes his courage is now put to the teft, and becomes immediately determined to conquer by violence or lofe his life in the attempt. This hafty refolve affords no moment to reflect upon the imperfections of our *own nature,* the daily inconfiftency of our proceedings, or the means by which they are excited or reftrained ; a total ftranger to the *fchool of philofophy,* and little read in the book of *refined fenfation,* he deals about him with whip and fpur moft unmercifully, till the animal (with perhaps a difpofition directly like his own) revolting ftill more at the feverity or inhumanity of the treatment, becomes outrageous, and by exertions of ftrength or ftratagem, difmounts his rider, or in a *retrogade motion* depofits him in a *ditch,* on one fide the rode or the other. The action is now renewed between *horfe and foot* in a different way,
the

the latter attacking the former with the utmost violence over the head and eyes, erroneously adopting AN IRICISM, to *bring him forward by driving him back :* This perpetual and severe discipline often rouses in the subject a certain kind of habitual callosity to every future intervention of tenderness, and renders him ever after incapable of becoming cheerfully obedient to what he considers his most inveterate enemy.

Some horses are also brought to a certain degree of starting exceedingly dangerous, by a similar and equally improper mode of treatment; for there can be no doubt but horses that are young, or have been but little used, must have some time, patience, care and attention bestowed to reconcile them to the *strange* and *numerous* objects upon a public road, before they can be expected to approach or pass them without sudden surprise and trouble. Indeed, the great variety and velocity of the different vehicles upon all the populous roads, but particularly round the metropolis, render it a matter of absolute wonder, how such an infinity of the highest mettled horses in the kingdom, should be

I 2

eternally

eternally paffing each other in crouds without thofe dreadful accidents fo natural to expect and fortunately fo little heard of.

It is really a matter of concern, that a cuf-tom fo inconfiderate and abfurd fhould ever have gained ground, as the practice of inftant-ly *beating* and *goading* a horfe upon his only method of expreffing a momentary and na-tural impulfe of fear, at any ftrange or un-common object that may come fuddenly upon him, or to which he may not have been accuftomed : In this, as the former cafe, a fimilar degree of feverity and cruel difplay of power are exerted by the major part of the *humane* and *enlightened* clafs before-mentioned ; for upon the horfe's firft ftart-ing, whether from fear or diflike, he in-ftantly receives a blow on the head with whip or ftick, accompanied with the very empha-tical impreffion of both fpurs, without allow-ing the poor animal a moment to recover from the firft furprife ; this repeated, conftitutes *a teremony* we have before explained, and totally deftroys the bafis of mutual confidence, that fhould be carefully preferved to infure the faithful

faithful fervices of one and the protection of the other.

Great inconveniencies arife from this un-juft and fevere method of treating horfes in general, where from blows indifcriminately dealt in paffion, the bones of the head, or the eyes, are irreparably injured by the fer-vant, and the real caufe never truly known to the mafter; feveral inftances having oc-curred within my own knowledge, of exfo-liations from the jaw bones, (with and with-out a diflodgement of teeth) fome of which I difcovered upon infpecting what the owners imagined to be a difeafe or canker in the mouth, and not till an examination of the bones of others after death; the greater part or all of which, I have no doubt, were pro-duced by blows with weapons very little cal-culated for *rods of correction.*

That there can be no doubt of horfes fuf-taining great injuries by thefe means, I have every reafon to believe, from numbers I have feen fall *inftantly* to the ground, upon receiving a blow feemingly flight and of no great force immediately behind the ear:

Among

Among those, my memory furnishes me with inftances of two that happened in the public parts of different large towns ; one paffionately inflicted by a brother of the faculty, the other by a fon of the church ; the laft of which was almoft accompanied with fo fingular a circumftance, that I cannot refift the temptation of a fhort digreffion to recite it.

Being a man of very low ftature, and engaged to preach (for an abfent friend) in an exceeding large church and high pulpit not a hundred miles from one of our univerfities, he delivered his text from that part of fcripture including the words, " *In a little time you fhall fee me, and in a little time you fhall not ;*" at this moment, the ftool upon which he ftood, to render himfelf confpicuous to the congregation, flipping from under him, rendered him not only inftantly *invifible,* but proved the words of his text to have been felected with the moft *prophetic infpiration,*

Leaving to the force of imagination the general confternation of his auditors and the confufion confusion of the preacher, I proceed to his additional mortification in the same town a short time after; where riding up to the door of his draper upon a favourite horse, and the horse very little used to the hurry of large towns, instantly started at some object within or without; when the little man, *in his warmth*, giving him a petulant blow upon the head, brought both horse and rider to the ground in the presence of twenty inhabitants, who having his former dilemma fresh in their memories, it doubly insured him the appendage of " A little time ye shall see me, and a little time ye shall not ;" which honourable distinction will, in all probability, accompany him to the grave, he being at present only in the prime of life.

From such remarks as I thought absolutely necessary to expose the cruelty of ill using horses, and demonstrate my invariable opinion, that *violence* and unjust severity, nine times out of ten, injures their tempers and confirms their vices; I come to such proof as may tend not only to obtain converts to *that opinion*, but to introduce a justification of my own ; viz. that horses of mild tempers and

pliable.

pliable difpofitions, may be brought to every
ftate of perfection by *gentle ufage* correfponding with their own frame of mind ; while,
on the contrary, the ferocity of the higheft
fpirited may be gradually fubdued by exertions of *fteady authority* and *perfevering forti-*
tude, blended with intervening acts of kind-
nefs and occafional encouragement, without
defcending to the moft unjuftifiable ill ufage,
tending only to excite invincible prejudice
and perpetual oppofition.

   The proofs upon which fuch opinion is
incontrovertibly founded, conftitute an experience of twenty years, in which time I have
attentively analized the tempers of horfes,
and the practical principles of *their breakers*
with as much fervency as the profeffional
abilities and medical knowledge of *Country*
Farriers, fo fully and repeatedly explained in
different parts of the former Volume. There
is a certain analogy in the practice of both ;
and *kill* or *cure* may be adopted by each for
his motto, without injury to either ; and with
much greater propriety than one of the fame
learned fraternity defined his employer's horfe
to be " *femper eadem,*" worfe and worfe ; or
                                                  the

the other, *Vivant Rex*, dead as a door nail, by G-d, Sir." Thefe flips are, however, to be charitably confidered fublime effufions of fancy, to which men of fuperior genius are juftly entitled, as laudably emerging from vulgar explanation, and fublimely foaring beyond the limits of common comprehenfion.

EXPERIENCE is, upon the foundation of the ancient adage, univerfally faid " *to make fools wife.*" To a little of that falutary experience I acknowledge myfelf indebted, and am not afhamed to confefs, that in the very early part of life, I became a temporary flave to cuftom, and creduloufly beftowed my premium of three guineas (exclufive of the keep) to have a colt rendered every thing *that was bad*, by the moft popular diftributor of equeftrian difcipline in the neighbourhood of my refidence; when after an abfence of fix weeks, the time fixed on neceffary to complete his education and render him a paragon of perfection, he was returned fo *caparifoned, bitted, cavifoned, martingaled*, and *cruppered*, that he feemed admirably decorated for the immediate adventures of a knight errant, the field day *charger*
of

of a general officer, or ready accoutred for the champion of England to make his public entry into Weftminfter Hall. My inftructions were, to ride him for fome time " *in his tackle,*" though he was as *well broke,* as *fteady, temperate* and *fafe* as any horfe in the kingdom." My very firft excurfion, however, convinced me of the honour and probity of this fcientific operator; for the colt was in poffeffion of every vice withouta fingle perfection in his favour, except a wonderful alacrity in *ftopping,* which he had the kindnefs to do unfolicited, at every *public houfe* upon the different roads for fome miles round; to all which he had been rotationally led, and daily placed for many hours in the ftable of *one or the other,* while his indefatigable tutor was, like " *friend Razor*" in the Upholfterer, conftantly getting drunk for the good of his country!

As I before faid, he was much worfe in qualities and condition than at his departure; but as the reward had been gradually drained during the time the fuppofed work was in hand, *purchafed experience* and *patient repentance* were the only remaining confolations.

lations. This mortifying impofition having excited no fmall degree of ftabularian emulation, I commenced *rough rider* to my own little eftablifhment, under the influence of juft refentment, determined to try the effect of frequent affociation, regular *perfonal* feeding, conftant exercife, and gentle treatment, to complete my purpofe ; which attempt having been crowned with the moft perfect fuccefs, and formed the bafis of all my future endeavours, I have never fince (a period of twenty-one years) condefcended to accept or reward the fervices of *breakers* or rough riders of any denomination for their *ineftimable* affiftance ; although in fome inftances I admit their utility, and acknowledge there are many, whofe merit and integrity are entitled to commendation and reward ; but their proportion is by no means equal to thofe pot valiant heroes, who take their *rides* and *potations* in ftrict fucceffion, upon the principle of *Pan in Midas*, who fays, "When I am moft rocky, I beft fit my faddle." This I can never be induced to doubt in oppofition to occular demonftration, as it is the general ftate in which I meet the *moft eminent profeffors* in every

part

part of the country; from whofe *fober* fyftem of inftruction their fubject muft certainly derive every neceffary advantage.

Without defcending to a tedious enumeration of the injuries colts in breaking, or
horfes in exercife, receive from pretended
breakers or worthlefs grooms under the effect
of intoxication, I return to the fubject of
thofe that are *refliff* or addicted to *ftarting*;
the general mifmanagement of which, I have
already defcribed without at all heightening
the picture to a degree of exaggeration, and
have now to add, that upon a well-founded
opinion of the inconfiftency of fuch fevere
treatment, I firft formed my determination
to encounter the cure of thofe defects, by a
method *directly oppofite*, whenever time fhould
afford me applicable opportunity.

It is, I muft acknowledge, fome little gratification of perfonal ambition, to have fucceeded fo well in a confirmation of the opinion I had indulged, refpecting the erroneous
and cruel treatment of horfes of fuch defcription; and with no trifling fatisfaction I
communicate the fact, of having been poffeffed

feffed at different times of three horfes incor-
rigibly *reftiff*, and as much fubject to that
dangerous failure of *ftarting* as any horfes in
the univerfe without exception. Thefe were
feparately purchafed with a perfect knowledge
of their defects, and at a price proportioned
to their deficiencies; each of the owners and
their fervants confidering themfelves in fuch
perpetual danger, that it was determined to
afford no farther chance of *a fracture for the
Surgeon* or a furvey for the *Coroner*; but to
difpofe of them at all events as *incurable*.
The horfes purchafed under fuch accumulation of difadvantages, (without arrogating
to myfelf a fuperiority in horfemanfhip or
courage) I reduced by a patient perfeverance
in the plan I have already laid down *(as
infallible)* to the moft pliable and beft con-
ditioned horfes I have ever had in poffeffion ;
ufing no other correction of feverity with
either *whip* or *fpur*, than juft fufficient to let
them be convinced I did not practice *lenity*
from the motive of *pufillanimity*, but to afford them the alternative of fubmitting to
treatment much more adapted to their own
eafe and fafety.

By

By this invariable preservation of temper and perseverance in discipline, I never found but little difficulty in effecting my purpose, not only in reducing them to unconditional submission, but in exciting so great an attachment from them, that their obedience and perfections in the field, or upon the road, rendered them objects of general request among my friends, at any equitable price I thought proper to fix them at. If I had, however, a single doubt remaining upon the propriety of this mode of treatment, a recent case has arisen to eradicate *a thousand* if they had existed; and left me in the most unsullied possession of an opinion, not to be relinquished upon the persuasion of any advocate for the violent measures I have so justly reprobated and so earnestly despise.

The instance so far exceeding all others I have seen, is of a blood horse now in my possession, and universally known to be one of the fleetest *in five* of the most fashionable popular hunts in the kingdom; this horse, when purchased, was perhaps the most *restiff*, *sullen*, and *refractory* ever brought into use; his figure and qualifications were neverthelesſ
so

fo palpably ftriking, they naturally excited every unremitting endeavour to reclaim him. The tafk, however, for the firft two or three weeks bore the moft unpromifing afpect ; no method that I could adopt, feemed to have the leaft effect upon the obduracy of his difpofition ; hardened to an almoft invincible fpirit of oppofition by former victories on his fide, and repeated ill ufage on the other, neither perfuafive encouragement nor violence could prevail on him to move a fingle yard forward but when it was perfectly his own pleafure; he would not only continually ftop in all paces, without the leaft obftacle or vifible caufe whatever, and continue his determination not to go at all forward for a great length of time, but perfevere in a retrogade motion an incredible diftance, with the ufual concomitants of *rearing, plunging,* and *kicking* to fo violent a degree, that numbers of a much more ferene and philofophic temper than myfelf, would have certainly proceeded in their refentment to the utmoft extremity, and fome time or other have left him *crippled* or *dead* upon the fpot. In this daily dilemma, it was the general opinion of intimate friends, and thofe who were conftant fpectators

fpectators of the *danger* I rode in for fome
weeks, that he was abfolutely not to be fubdued, and they pofitively advifed me to abandon the undertaking; but the inftinctive fpirit of attachment to that induftrious motto,
" PERSEVERE AND CONQUER," encouraged
me to continue my original plan, which I
have repeatedly explained and moft forcibly
recommend; for under that fyftem of fteady
and unremitting firmnefs, divefted of violence, and blended with intervening acts of
tender encouragement, he is become one of
the fteadieft and moft temperate hunters in the
field; though it is plainly perceptible by the
agitation fo conftantly difplayed in *the eye,
the ear, and action*, upon the approach of
every ftranger, that he had repeatedly experienced the fevere effects of bodily abufe and
ill ufage before he came into the *temperate
region* of my poffeffion.

These cafes are not introduced from any
motive of vanity, to blazon my own practice
with the ftamp of perfection in fafhionable
" feats of horfemanfhip," but to afford experimental, demonftrative, and incontrovertible
proof, (founded upon repeated perfonal trials

of

of time, patience and danger) that horse[s]
the moft perverfe, obftinate and refractory
are to be fubdued and rendered compleatly
tractable, with much more certainty, humanity, propriety and expedition, than by thofe
unjuftifiable acts of violence fo repeatedly
mentioned and accurately explained.

Convinced of this fact by the moft attentive obfervation, my mind is too fcru-
puloufly formed to admit of an alteration
in opinion ; and I cannot indulge the leaft
doubt, but the fubject will |undergo in
future a nicer decifion, by thofe gentlemen whofe opportunities have not been fufficiently numerous to afcertain the effect of
the different mode of treatment upon different fubjects to a critical degree of diftinction ; venturing alfo an additional belief, in
which I flatter myfelf moft obfervers will
coincide, that horfes originally *reftiff* or addicted to *fudden ftarting*, are continually
habituated in their vices by repeated ill ufage
of fervants and the perpetual transfer from
one owner to another, under all the difadvantage, prejudice, and refentment inflicted
upon *a bad name*, without the lucky chance

of once falling into patient and proper hands
to effect the work of reformation.

S H O E I N G

IS a matter of fo much importance,
that it cannot be too clearly explained, or
too generally underftood, confequently creates no furprife that fo many writers have
condefcended to offer their fentiments upon
a fubject of fuch magnitude ; but it is to be
ferioufly regretted, thofe opinions have been
fubmitted to public infpection in fo remote a way, as applies much more to the
profeffional conception of individuals than
the ftandard of general comprehenfion.

The various differtations upon fhoeing, or
difeafes of the feet, have been in general
too fublime in their language and too much
interfperfed with anatomical difquifition and
technical jargon, to acquire public patronage and commendation ; to fuch inconfiftency
alone may perhaps be juftly attributed their
confignment to oblivion fo foon after publication. A minute and fcientific inveftigation or anatomical defcription of all the correfponding parts, their actions and effects,

cannot.

cannot be the moft proper and confiftent method of being clearly underftood by the very clafs or claffes of people particularly interefted in the explanation. Ruftic *Farriers* and uneducated *grooms cannot*, and GENTLEMEN *will not*, embark in the dull and difagreeable tafk of theoretic or practical diffection, to difcover the feat and appropriation of the *tendo Achilles*, or the articulation of the *coronary bone*; nor do I confider it more neceffary for a gentleman to pafs through a ftudy of this kind to afcertain a proper *conditional* method of ordering his horfes to be fhod, than to go through a courfe of anatomical lectures and phyfical enquiries, becaufe, like the reft of mankind, he is fubject to daily indifpofition.

Abftrufe ftudy upon fo plain a fubject can never be expected from all the claffes fo immediately concerned, it therefore becomes the province of the writer, to reduce his inftructions to fuch concife undifguifed explanation, and mode of plain reafoning *on one fide*, as may require no uncommon powers of comprehenfion *on*

K 2

the

the other. Authors are too frequently vain of their own abilities, and seem to believe too much matter cannot be introduced (however extraneous or digreffive) to give their works the appearance of elaborate ftudy and profound erudition; lofing the fubject in an affected fublimity of diction, without adverting to the great numbers who either wish to acquire information by every poffible means where the *trouble of reading* can be avoided, or to obtain the purport of their medical refearches by the moft fuperficial and leaft expenfive enquiry.

The various animadverfions of different writers under this head, are evidently too clofely wrapped in the veil of obfcurity, and feem purpofely addreffed much more to the anatomical judgement of the fcientific Artift and operative Farrier, than to the underftandings of the many, by whom we are to fuppofe it fhould be *equally underftood.* An elegant arrangement of words, and ambiguity of expreffion, may conftitute a loftinefs of ftile more pleafing to the gentleman, or the fcholar, delighting in a judicious difplay of polifhed periods; but

in

in the prefent inftance is required, fuch eafy flow of plain defcriptive matter, as becomes perfectly applicable to the infe- rior capacities proportionally interefted in its effects, who have not the leaft right to be excluded their fhare of knowledge, for the oftentatious introduction of pedantic phrafeology.

Such connected chain of ufeful informa- tion, divefted of obfcure references to re- mote confiderations, (that ferve only to erect one myftery upon the bafis of ano- ther) muft certainly prove much more ap- plicable to the intentional purport of com- mon conception and general improvement, than the many laboured differtations whofe titles promife *fo much*, and whofe learned contents communicate *fo little*, at leaft, to be generally underftood: Under the influence of this impreffion, I have ever confidered fuch concife, plain, intelligent advice, as will enable every gentleman, fportfman, or tra- veller, to perceive the neceffity of adapting the mode of fhoeing to the fhape of his horfe's foot, and the manner of his going, is all that can be required; to prevent bow-

K 3

ing

ing implicit obedience to the felf-fufficient dictation of every *rural Vulcan*, who in general fpeaks fuch " an infinite deal of nothing," that it is equally difficult to underftand as to be underftood.

Previous to farther progrefs upon a fub-ject we will endeavour to treat with great plainnefs and perfpicuity, it becomes un-avoidably neceffary to take a flight furvey of the inconfiftent ground-work, upon which the fabric of fuch publications have been raifed; as we may, perhaps, have occafion to introduce fome few obfervations of prac-tical remarks upon the propriety of their recommendations, which fhall neverthelefs be produced with all poffible delicacy to the different writers, wifhing by no means to irritate their feeling in the fupport of an oppofite opinion, where an incumbent duty renders the inculcation indifpenfible.

The inconfiderate career of fome pens, and the invincible *cacoethes fcribendi* of others, compel the involuntary tafk of dif-quifition, to prevent the ill effect of lite-rary impofition, or mifreprefentation, upon
the

the credulity and inexperienced judgment of individuals; who are in general, *particularly the uncultivated claſſes,* (by far the moſt numerous) diſpoſed to believe every thing ſanctioned with the authority of the preſs and the name of the Printer bears the incontrovertible ſtamp of infallibility. Under the influence of this reflection, and to prove the ſtrict juſtice of the aſſertion, it becomes directly in point to ſtate ſuch inconſiſtencies as evidently ariſe in retroſpection. A writer of the preſent day confidently tells us in his title page, he is " an experienced Farrier of fifty years practice," and promiſes (according to cuſtom) a great deal more information and inſtruction than he ever condeſcended to perform. He then leads you through two hundred pages of dull uninteresting *anatomical deſcriptive,* obliquely copied from the elaborate work of GIBSON; interlards the remaining hundred and ſeventy pages with the almoſt obſelete preſcriptive parts of the ancient Syſtem of Farriery, (ſlightly varied to evade the charge of direct plagiariſm) without the coinage of a *new thought,* or the leaſt indicated knowledge

K 4

ledge of a *new medicine*. The utility of
bark, opium, antimony, and mercury, thofe
grand fupporters of the MATERIA MEDICA,
feem almoft unknown to him ; and that great
bafis of external application in modern
practice, with its accumulation of valuable
properties, the SATURNINE EXTRACT,
he has never once given proof of the moft
fuperficial acquaintance with. But what
renders it ftill more extraordinary is, that
out of fo great a number of pages he has
thought proper to beftow, upon the fubject of *fhoeing, and all the diforders, accidents, or infirmities, to which the feet are
liable,* twelve only, including his long and
inoffenfive prefcripts for their mitigation or
cure. However, as the circulation of the
book has been too contracted and infignificant to gratify the wants, or eftablifh the
reputation of the writer, it will be but *an
act of charity* to contract the remarks *alfo,*
fubmitting both to their inevitable oblivion.

Another of not only longer ftanding, but
much greater eftimation, has condefcended
to afford a few more " REFLECTIONS UPON
SHOEING

Shoeing Horses;" but, exclusive of its being a confessed translation (and consequently entitled to little more respect than *hear-say evidence* in a court of justice) it is so replete with mechanical principles and mathematical reasoning; so intersperfed with abstruse references and technical allusions to certain *bones* and *tendons*, their *motions* and *effects*, that I cannot reconcile the description as at all applicable to the intellectual capacities of those mostly concerned in the operative or superintending part of the process.

A third has produced what he denominated " A Treatise on the Diseases and Lameness of Horses, with a proper Method of *Shoeing in general*; but whether from a want of stability in his own disposition (or what other motive I know not) he soon took a formal leave of the principal subject, and entertained his readers with a dance through Turkey, the desarts of Arabia, and a comparative survey of the whole animal creation; ornamenting almost every page with various *Latin quotations*, as an excitement to the general improvement of
all

all parties interefted in the *explanatory* parts of his work.

This author, in the early part of his tract, fays, "If you pretend to have your horfe fhod according to your own mind, it is a general faying among thefe men, that they do not want to be taught." This very acknowledgment of his juftifies the neceffity of recommending to the remembrance of every gentleman, fportfman, or traveller, that he is, *in the bufinefs of fhoeing,* only the imaginary main fpring in the *operative part;* and that his inclination or directions become unavoidably dependant upon the will of another. That this remark may be divefted of its paradoxical appearance, let it be underftood how very much the *fafety,* propriety, and excellence of manual execution depend upon the well-timed liberality of THE GENTLEMAN; or, in farther illuftration of a paffage that may favor too much of *ambiguity* to thofe whofe pecuniary pulfations render it difficult of comprehenfion, it is almoft incredible how very much occafional judicious interpofitions of *good beer,* (or the means to obtain it) with the fubordinate operator, improves,

to

to a certainty, the fyftem of " SHOEING IN GENERAL," through every part of England.

The mechanical world at large ftand in no need of information, that in all climates, regions, countries, and counties, there are (paffing under the denomination of *gentlemen)* poffeffors of horfes, too mean and mercenary ever to be *obeyed,* farther than they can command by the inceffant fufpicion and perfonal fatigue of ocular demonftration; whofe very *fervants,* as well as *tradefmen,* juftly hold them in fo much deteftation, and whofe conduct is fo *inconfiftently confiftent,* that it ferves only to encreafe the general odium of their characters, (with the additional mortification of feeling the weight of the opprobrium) without the power or inclination to retrieve them.

This univerfal refentment extends itfelf, in its effects, to his moft trifling concerns; the fame diflike and indifference that follow him in all other refpects, attend him in this; the fignificant appellation of " *a d——d bad one* " is equitably beftowed upon him by the domeftics under his own roof,

and

and re-echoed from *fervant to fmith, and fmith to fervant;* while the poor animal becomes the fubject of paffive obedience; for whether *well* or *ill fhod, pricked* or *lamed,* is a matter of indifference to all parties except the owner, who being thus acknowledged fo defpicable a character, no one feels for his difquietude or misfortunes, but exultingly exclaims, that what's too *bad* for another is too *good* for him.

Such characters as thefe are not the prolific effect of a fertile imagination, but exact pictures of *objects* the produce of every foil. No gratification of ambition, no perfonal oftentation, can be indulged in the prefent difcrimination, by arraigning the difgraceful want of liberality in others, or vainly endeavouring to extol my own: It is, however, matter of the moft unfullied exultation, that fuch accufation has never been known to reach the hofpitable hall of a SPORTSMAN'S HABITATION; their univerfally admitted generofity (calculating upon the principle of felf-prefervation) ftands much more in need of the *curb* than the *fpur,* the general tenor of every

pursuit

parfuit leaving them totally exculpated from the bare fufpicion of being included in the " *beggarly* defcription."

Taking leave, therefore, of that part of the fubject as can but ill accord with the feelings of thofe who may become perfonally affected by fo faithful a reprefentation of their domeftic !penury; I beg permiffion to recommend for their deliberative imitation, a part of my invariable practice for a feries of more than twenty years. This has always been, to let the manual operator (or *journeyman*, whom I ever confidered the *main fpring* of the machine) enjoy fome pecuniary compenfation, in addition to the profeffional emolument of the mafter, not more from a confcientious conviction of its being greatly merited by the trouble, care, and danger of fhoeing high fpirited and refractory horfes, than experimental demonftration, that GENEROSITY, founded upon the *bafis of equity*, will inevitably infure its own reward. This is at leaft a leffon I have every right to inculcate, when I can affirm with the ftricteft veracity, I have never had a horfe fuftain

tain the most trifling injury under the hands of the SMITH, nor ever a horse *plated* but what proved a *winner*.

The trifling attention, the humane bene-faction of a cooling beverage to allay thirst in the exceffive heat of summer, or the falutary interpofition of an invigorating cor-dial to encounter the extreme feverity of froft or fnow in winter, are offices of kind-nefs that in their vifible effects upon the *hand* and *hammer*, infure, beyond a doubt, the fafety of the horfe and the reputation of the owner. The philanthropic influence of " doing as you would be done unto," is repaid with the moft flattering intereft, the fame care and attention beftowed upon the feet in fhoeing, are extended in general tendernefs to the fafety of the whole frame, upon all other profeffional occafions; if refractory or vicious, he is foothed by *kind-nefs*, not provoked by *violence*; in fhort, whatever fatigue enfues, whatever difficulty occurs, the execution is cheerfully com-pleated, with a retrofpective reference to the perfevering hofpitality of the MASTER; who living in an unvaried fcene of uni-

niat   verfal

verfal benevolence amidft his happy domeftics, enjoys the very anticipation of his
wifhes in the cheerful fervices of a long
lift of *old* and *faithful* dependents.

. A contraft in character fo exceedingly
common, that it may be found in almoft
every parifh in the kingdom, is perhaps
well worthy the attention of thofe who
may be at all interefted in the defcription,
or their different effects. The conftant ill
ufage and violent abufe of horfes, either *ti-*
mid, vicious, or *refractory,* under the hands
of the operator, is a matter of fufficient no-
toriety to every man who has had occafion
to fuperintend their practice; fuch cruelties
require not to be fought after in remote cor-
ners by fcrutinizing curiofity, they meet the
eye of the TRAVELLER daily in the moft
public fituations. No judicious obferver, no
old groom or *young fmith,* need be reminded
what an infinity of fine and valuable horfes
go through a tedious tafk of mifery in repeated *bleedings, mercurial purges, rowels,*
and courfe of *alteratives,* for defects or
difeafes in the eyes, originating only in the
cruel hand and heavy hammer of the SMITH,
with

with the emphatical accompaniment of
" *stand still and be d——d to ye,*" when
shifting and uneasy under the operation of
shoeing ; a circumstance that during a certain season of the year, is frequently occasioned by *flies only,* and consequently to be
removed with very little trouble either to
the animal, or his *more inveterate perse-
cutor.*

This delineation may serve as an epitome
of the many injuries sustained from similar
acts of injustice, the true causes of which
are never discovered or known but to the
inhuman perpetrators : From severe blows
with instruments of this kind (as hammer,
pinchers, blood-stick, &c.) frequently originate lameness in various parts, tumours,
formations of matter, wounds, exfoliations,
with others too numerous and probable for
enumeration ; all or either of which, are
generally attributed to a different cause, or
defect in the constitution, and treated accordingly. Injuries to the *eyes* and dislodge-
ment of the *teeth,* are, however, among the
most common evils of this kind ; which are
in general tolerably reconciled to the too
great

great credulity of the owner, by the plaufible fiction of the experienced adept in impofition, who is always prepared to report
one the effect of a *kick*, the other a *bite*.
Dangerous as thefe practices are to horfes of
any age or qualifications, they are doubly fo
to young ones; for a degree of feverity and
ill ufage at their firft and fecond fhoeings,
very frequently fixes in the difpofition an
habitual averfion to SMITHS, and a reluctance
in approaching their *fhops*, never after to be
obliterated by any means whatever; and however opinions may clafh upon the fubject of
extreme feverity to horfes, I fhall continue
to perfevere in the truth of my former affertion,——if they are innately *timid, vicious*, or
reftive, unconditional violence alone will never
make them better.

Having found it unavoidable to introduce
remarks that are not only evidently connected with, but neceffary to ufher in the
fubject, we now proceed to fuch fuperficial
knowledge of the operative part, as it is
abfolutely requifite every perfon fhould be
in poffeffion of, who wifhes to underftand,
and retain the power to direct a method of

VOL. II. L fhoeing,

fhoeing, beft adapted to the foot and action of his own horfe. I never confidered it at all neceffary that a gentleman, fportfman, tradefman, or traveller, is to commence *blackfmith* in theory, and go through the rudiments of the trade to promote his intention ; that has been hitherto the fyftematic mode of tuition : But when it is confidered how very few will enter a wide field of abftrufe ftudy, to comprehend what he *is* told is a proper method of *fhoeing his horfe*, it can create no furprife that it has been attended with fo little fuccefs.

My conception of the neceffary knowledge is unequivocally this : Although every SMITH in profeffional etiquette may be deemed an *artift*, I defy the force of *logic itfelf* to render every artift a *conjurer* ; and as there muft inevitably remain among the collateral defcendants from VULCAN (as in moft other profeffions) fome *prodigies of brightnefs*, who, incapable of diftinguifhing right from wrong, *fhoe one horfe as they fhoe another*, or, in plainer Englifh, *fhoe all alike* ; fuch difcrimination becomes palpably ufeful, as will enable the owners to give conditional

onal directions for the ease and safety of his horse, without relying entirely upon those who will frequently be found to possess little or no judgment at all.

The greater part of those writers who have favoured the public with a communication of their sentiments upon this subject, seem extravagantly fond of an idea borrowed from antiquity, and transferred from one to another, upon the practicability of horses travelling the road, and doing their constant work without any shoeing at all: Such œconomical plan may be admirably calculated for the *theoretical journey* of some literary speculatist, up two or three pair of stairs in a remote corner of the metropolis; but I will venture to affirm, no such excursion can take place of any duration, without material injury to thee HOOF, unless to the *high bred horses of authors*, many of whom enjoy their journies, as Bajazet enjoyed his cruelty, only " IN IMAGINATION."

One of these (OSMER) has introduced his remarks with the following rhapsodical expostulation:

" When

" When time was young, when the earth was in a ſtate of nature, and turnpike roads as yet were not, the horſe needed not the aſſiſtance of this artiſt; for the divine artiſt had taken care to give his feet ſuch defence as it pleaſed him; and who is weak enough to ſuppoſe his wiſdom was not ſufficient to the purpoſe in ſuch a ſtate ?''

He then proceeds to juſtify an opinion, that horſes are adequate to their different ſervices in a ſtate of *nature* without the offi-cious obtruſions of *art*; venturing to affirm that they " will travel even upon the turn-pike roads about London, without injury to their feet." I avail myſelf of the preſent opening to diſclaim every idea of attacking the remarks or opinions of others, from a motive of intentional oppoſition, or to in-dulge a vein of ſatire, that aſſertions ſo cy-nically ſingular and extraordinary naturally excite; and ſhall therefore introduce upon the preſent occaſion no other reflection than a certain ſenſation of ſurpriſe, that he did not inſinuate the palpable ſuperfluity or lux-ury of *ſhoes and ſtockings* to the natives of our own country, particularly when even the

fair

fair sex of many neighbouring kingdoms convince us they can walk *equally upright* without.

In farther confirmation of the belief he wishes to establish, he says, " we may every day see horses, mares, and colts running about upon all sorts of ground unshod, and uninjured in their feet." This is certainly a truth too universally known even to be questioned; but by no means to be so far strained in its construction as to be rendered applicable (in a comparative view) to the state of working horses upon hard or stony roads, where the constant friction in riding, or the *fulcrum* in drawing, must inevitably prove injurious, if not totally destructive to the foot in general; producing *sand-cracks, thrush, bruises of the frog, formations of matter*, and other infirmities, as is very frequently the case, (when a shoe has been for some time cast unobserved by the rider;) constituting a blemish or defect in the subject never to be retrieved. Mares and colts, or horses turned out to grass without shoes, are generally kept upon low, moist, or marshy

L 3 ground,

ground, admirably adapted to preferve the
foot in a growing ftate of perfection; the
cafe is exceedingly different, and will bear no
parallel with horfes of the above defcription ;
nor can I hefitate to believe, but the abfolute
neceffity of fubftantially guarding the foot,
is too well eftablifhed by immemorial experience, to be at all fhaken by the introduction of any *new* opinions upon that part of
the fubject.

I muft, to avoid a mifconception of my
purpofe, before I proceed, confefs my obli-
gation as an individual, to the memories
of thofe gentlemen who have formerly attended to and written upon this head, with
a defire to improve it for the promotion of a
general good; and am forry a total want of
paffive pliability in my own pen, will not permit me to adhere to the " *good old cuftom*"
of implicitly tranfmitting to fucceeding gene-
rations, the immaculate purity of *their* dic-
tations, without prefuming to introduce an
opinion of my *own*.

" Learn to do well by others' harm" is
an axiom of too much excellence to be ob-

3   literated

literated from a memory replete with obfervant advantages arifing from reflection.   If
I could become fo fubfervient to the fafhionable impulfe of literary ambition as to expect to be generally read, and after fuch
reading to be generally underftood, I might
enjoy much pleafure in going over the defcriptive confirmation of the *bones, tendons,*
the *inner flefhy,* and the *outer horny fole,* the
frog, and *cruft* or *hoof,* with their different
appropriations ; but having the moft indifputable reafon to believe, *that very abftrucity
of reafoning,* and myfterious introduction of
technical terms, have in a great degree prevented the reading of publications upon this
fubject, I fhall (in earneft hope of laying juft
claim to fuperior attention) defcend, like the
orator in one of the celebrated Foote's co-
medies, " to the vale of *common fenfe,* that I
may be the better underftood."

It has been the fecondary confideration
of thefe fpeculative writers, or theoretical
fportfmen, (fuppofing a perfeverance in the
cuftom of fhoeing not to be abolifhed upon
the power of their perfuafions) to propagate and re-echo a doctrine equally abfurd,

L 4   tending

tending to what they *pretend to believe,* a proportional reformation in some part of the operation; viz. " That the *sole* and *frog* of a horse's foot need never be *pared at all.*" To take up as little of the reader's time as the nature of the observation will admit, I shall very much contract what I wish to introduce more at large upon the inconfiftency of the declaration; particularly, as thefe *refinements* feem brought forward more from a fcarcity of matter, neceffary to complete their arrangement of pages for the prefs, than the leaft probable utility to be derived from remarks fo erroneous in their formation.

Says the author before-mentioned, in continuation of his affertions, borrowed from *La Foffe,* " There is another reafon equally obvious; which is, that the wifdom of the Creator intended this outer fole, and its obduracy, as a natural and proper defence to the inner fole, which lies immediately under the other, between that and the bone of the foot." He then proceeds, " If it be afked, what becomes of the fole when not pared ?

pared? It dries, feparates, and fcales away."
In concife reply to this fublime juftification, and *very fimple* explanation, I fhould
in any converfation with the writer, if he
had not paffed " that bourne from whence
no traveller returns," have folicited a greater
degree of candour in his opinion; Whether the *nails* were not furnifhed to our
own frames by the " wifdom of the Creator
as a natural and proper defence" to parts
of the moft exquifite fenfibility? And
whether the exuberant fuperflux in conftant
growth was never to be reduced to the
ftandard of mediocrity, till every individual
of the human fpecies became a *voluntary
Nebuchadnezzar*; becaufe, upon the opinions
of LA FOSSE, OSMER, and *others*, it would
be the greateft prefumption to fuppofe
" the divine artift" had left in any part of
his works the leaft room for rectification?

We might certainly introduce with propriety, a fucceffion of fimilies perfectly in
point to render the idea ridiculous; refifting
however, the great temptation to animadvert
upon palpable abfurdities, we come to the
proof

proof of its " *drying, separating,* and *scaling away*." The fact is not literally so, as may be corroborated by any judicious observer accustomed to examine the feet of horses with the degree of accuracy and nice distinction, necessary to *justify* or *disprove* any opinion that may be promulgated for public investigation or improvement. It is a matter too well known to admit of momentary cavil, that the foot by being permitted to remain too long in its natural state without reduction, acquires in its several parts the appearance of deformity; the hoof grows *long, narrow,* and *weak*; the *sole,* as he says, *separates,* (but in part only) and comes away in PARTIAL SCALES, leaving a rough, hard, uneven surface of *cavities* and *projections*; the frog becoming bruised, ragged, and putrefied, even to different degrees of lameness. This being the exact representation of a foot left to growth in a rude and unimproved state, the propriety or impropriety of judiciously paring *each part*, to promote a corresponding firmness, and preserve the necessary uniformity, can never become the subject of disputation, but among those whose intellectual faculties are

absorbed

abforbed in fuch an abundant flow of *imaginary matter*, as to render practical refearches and ocular demonftration too infignificant for the condefcending enquiries of fuperior underftandings.

Previous to a defcription of the different kinds of feet, at leaft the quality or texture of their formation, and the mode of SHOEING beft adapted to each ; a few words may be properly introduced upon the many horfes rendered *temporary cripples* by the injudicious or improper mode of forming or fetting a fhoe, without a relative confideration to the *fhape* or *make* of the foot, or the *fize* and *action* of the horfe. What renders the circumftance ftill more extraordinary is, that this error in judgment fo conftantly happens without the leaft difcovery by either owner or operator in their frequent furveys and tedious confultations; and I am the more ftrengthened in my confirmation of this fact, by the repeated inftances, where the ceremonies of embrocating with thofe *Vulcanian fpecifics*, origanum and turpentine, have been perfevered in

in (even to the acts of BLISTERING and
ROWELLING) till by my defire *the fhoe has
been taken off,* when the caufe has been
inftantly difcovered and immediately removed.

This is a circumftance, that I doubt
not has fo frequently happened in the remembrance of every reader of experience,
it can ftand in no need of farther illuftration; we therefore proceed to fuch defcription of the *exterior parts* immediately concerned in the operation of fhoeing, as upon
a fuperficial furvey meet the eye of every
infpector. Thefe are, firft, the *bottom* or
lower edge of the HOOF, furrounding the
whole extremity of the foot, not only as a
fafeguard and general defence againft external injuries, but is the direct part to
which the fhoe is fcientifically fixed, to effect the purpofes for which it was generally intended. Secondly, the *horny* or
OUTER SOLE, covering the entire bottom of
the foot, except the FROG, which is fitu-
ate in the center, (paffing in a longitudinal
direction from *heel to toe*) and forms by its
elafticity the fulcrum, or expanding bafis

of

of the tendon upon which the very action of the horfe depends.

Thefe are the external parts appearing upon the furface, that prefent themfelves to the fpectator, and conftitute in general all that he is fuppofed or required to know; remote confiderations and operative confequences appertaining much more to the profeffional knowledge of the ARTIST than any acquired information of the OWNER.

Perfectly convinced that every man may judicioufly fuperintend, or properly direct the fhoeing of his horfe, in a manner evidently adapted to his *foot, fize, weight, purpofe,* and *manner of going,* without the ill-according intervention of an abftrufe ftudy very little attended to, (however elaborately urged) I forbear impofition upon public patience, by any attempt to introduce an imitation or oblique copy of anatomical defcriptive, fo accurately delineated and defcribed in the copper-plates and references of GIBSON and BARTLET, with, I am forry to fay, *fo little fuccefs*; if I may be allowed to explain, by an opinion that the

4

Farriers

Farriers themselves, a very inferior proportion excepted, seem to have imbibed no additional knowledge in equeſtrian anatomy, from ſtudies ſo laudably exerted and clearly explained.

We come next to an explanation of the different kinds of feet, as they appear in different ſubjects in their natural ſtate. Theſe may be defined under three diſtinct heads ; the ſhort, ſound, *black*, ſubſtantial hoof ; the ſhallow, long, weak, *white*, *brittle* hoof ; and the deep, lax, *porous*, *ſpongy* hoof. Of theſe, the firſt is ſo evidently ſuperior, that unleſs by improper or unfair treatment, it hardly ever becomes the ſubject of diſeaſe. The next is carefully to be avoided in the purchaſe if poſſible, not only on account of their being more ſubject to *corns* than any other, but indicative in a great degree of conſtitutional delicacy in either horſe or mare, they not being ſo well enabled to bear hard work or conſtant fatigue. The laſt of the three is ſo equally inferior to the firſt, that from a variety of cauſes it is frequently productive of inceſſant attention, anxiety, diſeaſe, and lameneſs.

Having

Having taken a view of the kinds of feet that conftantly pafs through the hands of the SMITH in his daily practice; and knowing the various ftates and forms in which they become fubject to his infpection; it is abfolutely impoffible, in all that ever *has been* written, or *can be* advanced, to lay down certain and invariable rules for the exact management of *this*, or the direct treatment of *that particular foot*, without a conditional reference to the judicious eye and difcretional hand of the OWNER or OPERATOR. It muft prove palpably clear to every enlightened enquirer, that no opinion or directions *ftrictly infallible* can be communicated through the medium of the prefs, applicable to every particular purpofe, without proportional contribution from the judgment of the parties concerned, to give the ground work of *conditional information* its proper effect.

Such inftructions, however *accurately defcribed*, muft unavoidably remain fubject to contingent deviations, regulated entirely by the ftate of the foot and circumftances of the cafe;

cafe; in a multiplicity of which, fo many unexpected variations occur, as render one fixed mode of fhoeing abfolutely impractica-ble with *every kind of horfe*, notwithftanding what may have been hitherto advanced from SUPPOSED HIGH AUTHORITY to the con-trary.

There are, neverthelefs, fome general rules in the proper fyftem of fhoeing and preferv-ing the feet, not to be eafily miftaken by folly or perverted by ignorance, that fhall be fub-mitted to confideration before we take leave of the fubject before us; previous to which, fome part of M. LA FOSSE's obfervations, fo ftrenuoufly recommended by BARTLET, become well worthy the attention of every gentleman or fportfman, who may wifh to affift his judgment in the enquiry, and enable himfelf to decide *impartially*, upon the pro-priety or impropriety of having his horfe fhod upon principles that have ftood hitherto incon-troverted, from a fear (I fufpect) of arraigning authorities, the dread of whofe names may have deterred many practitioners of eminence from fo defirable a purpofe.

I have

I have more than once afferted my determination to interfere as little as poffible with the opinions or inftructions of former writers, but where it became unavoidably neceffary to eftablifh an oppofite opinion, or corroborate a fact. It is a matter of fome furprife that authors of eminence, who are naturally fuppofed to be " armed at all points," fhould be fo incautioufly off their guard, as to contradict themfelves in the very act and emulation of conveying tuition to others. I have given a moft ftriking inftance of this error in my former volume, upon the inadvertency of Os-MER, who repeatedly fays, with the *greateft confidence* and *feeming belief,* " Tendons are unelaftic bodies ;" and frequently, in the fame or the very next page, tells you, ": *the tendon was elongated.*" I believe fuch affertion is of a complection too paradoxical to require from me the moft trifling elucidation.

Paffing over this *privilege of authors* with no other remark than bare remembrance, I come directly to the analyzation of as palpable a profeffional contradiction broached by LA FOSSE, and given to the public by BART-LET, in the true fpirit of implicit and

M enthufiaftic

enthufiaftic obedience. Thefe Gentlemen have in fucceffion, after going over (as before obferved) a great deal of unneceffary ground totally unintelligible to the *fporting world*, endeavoured to convince us, that *paring the fole or frog*, is not only unneceffary, but abfolutely prejudicial; for, fay they, to eftablifh a credulous confirmation of their erroneous conjecture, " if you pare away the fole or frog in any degree, the more you pare, the farther you take from the ground the fupport of the tendon, which fo entirely depends upon the elafticity of the frog." If any one perfon living could be found fo unexpectedly ignorant as to pare the *foot partially* (that is, all behind and none before) fuch effect might probably enfue; but furely no rational obferver will attempt to deny or difprove a palpable demonftration, that all parts of the foot being *equally pared*, (that is, the HOOF, SOLE, and FROG) the centre of fupport and action muft be ftill the fame.

But was it really as they have faid; if what they have fo *learnedly advanced* was literally and juftly true, what do they immediately do after this judicious and dicta-

9

torial

torial decifion ? Why, ftrongly recommend, with the full force of theoretic perfuafion, the introduction of a mode of fhoeing *directly contradictory* to the opinion juft recited ; that may be perfectly adapted to and coincide with the fentiments of any writer in the act of amufing *himfelf,* employing the *Printer,* and deceiving the *Public* ; but can never be brought into general practice, without perpetual hazard to the horfe, and imminent danger to the rider. This is fo perfectly clear, that I will go very far beyond bare literary affertion, and be bound to ftake both property and profeffional reputation, upon the certain failure of their improved propofition of fhoeing, with what they call their half-moon fhoe, with all its boafted advantages. A long chain of remarks in oppofition is by no means neceffary, a very concife and candid inveftigation will afford ample proof of their having reconciled (in compliment to their patient readers) as palpable contradictions in defcription as Os-MER, whofe " unelaftic tendon" was immediately after " elongated."

You are given to underftand (as I have

before obferved) that in their opinion, if you
pare the *fole* or *frog*, you prevent the heel
of the horfe from coming into conftant contact with the ground; and the tendon is deprived of the elaftic affiftance of the frog
to promote its expanfion and contraction.
This is at leaft the exact purport of their
defcription, if not given in the very fame language, and is very well entitled to the deliberate attention of thofe who wifh to underftand
accurately the ftate of the tendon (or back
finews) when in the *Stabularian tongue* they
are faid to be " *let down.*"

Such a paring and hollowing out of the
heel as they feem to defcribe, muft be a moft
unmerciful deftruction of parts, and what I
believe can feldom happen in the prefent age,
unlefs in the remote and leaft improved parts
of the kingdom. Concluding, however, they
took only a conjectural furvey of this matter, I muft beg leave to obferve, that immediately after reprobating the idea of raifing
the frog from the ground by *paring*, they
ftrenuoufly recommend a much more certain method of producing *the very evil* they
tell you they wifh *to prevent.* And this by
raifing

raising all the fore part of the foot, with
" the half-moon shoe, set on to the middle of the hoof," not only forming an irregular and preternatural surface, but (by a
want of length and support at the heel) constituting an unavoidable chance of relaxing the
sinews in the perpetual probability of their
being extended beyond the *elastic power* pre-
scribed by nature.

This difference of opinion becomes so immediately connected with a particular passage
in my former volume (upon the subject of
" *strains*,") that it is absolutely necessary to
quote a few lines for the better comprehension of the case before us; for I have there
said, " To render this idea so clear that
it cannot be misunderstood, let us suppose
that a horse is going at his rate, and in so
doing his toe covers a prominence, or the
edge of one, where the heel *has no support*, it consequently extends the tendons
beyond the distance afforded by nature, and
instantly continues what is called a letting
down of the back sinews," a circumstance
that constantly happens upon the turf in run-

ning for a heat, and the horfe is then faid to
have " broken down."

This defcription comes fo directly in point
with the fhape and ftate of the horfe's foot
in *their mode of fhoeing*, that the horfe muft
be at all times liable to fudden lamenefs,
and more particularly at the rifing of *every
hill*, where his foot would be exactly in
the fituation by which I have defcribed ftrains
to be acquired. Every Reader at all acquainted with, or having even a *tolerable
idea* of the anatomical ftructure of the leg
and foot, by taking a comparative view of
the mode of fhoeing recommended, and the
evident manner of fuftaining an injury in the
back finews, as they are termed, will be
fufficiently enabled to decide upon the *confiftency* of the propofed plan, and, I flatter
myfelf, enough convinced of the danger, to
coincide with me in opinion, that a horfe
fhod in this manner, to cover a hilly country either in *a journey* or *the chace*, muft
inevitably fall *dead lame* from a relaxation
of the tendinous parts; or, even in a low
flat country, become fo exceedingly weary
from a want of proper fupport for the heel,
that

that he could never be able to go through a fecond day's fatigue without an alteration in his favour.

Establishing this as a fact not to be controverted by the fallacious effect of speculative rumination, and perfectly convinced neither entertainment nor utility can be derived from farther tedious explanatory remarks and observations upon the inconveniences of fuch mode of fhoeing, as well as the numerous difficulties not to be furmounted if inadvertently encountered; I fhall only flightly infinuate the abfolute *impoffibility* of hunting or travelling (particularly in the rainy feafons) in various hilly or chalky parts of the kingdom, without the accumulated probabilities of lamenefs to the horfe, continual danger to the rider, and the inevitable certainty of bruifing the heel and frog to a degree of difeafe, which muft prove the refulting evil even upon the flatteft and beft turnpikes; but in the rough and ftony roads, or ftrong and dry hard clays, fuch events may be expected as totally unavoidable.

Bidding adieu to a mode of fhoeing calcu-
M 4   lated

lated only for the foft and artificial floor-
ing of a FRENCH RIDING SCHOOL, we
come to fuch confiderations as are adapted
to the ftate of our own roads, the cuftoms
of our country, and the intellectual faculties
of thofe to whofe fcientific fkill the mallea-
bility of the metal, the important ufe of the
butteris, the judicious formation of the fhoe,
and the equally decifive direction of the nail,
are univerfally entrufted. Adverting for a
moment to the before-mentioned allufion to
OSMER's obfervation upon thefe men, who
fay, " they do not want to be taught," it
is very natural to fuppofe, from the profeffional knowledge *they fhould have acquired* by
ftrict attention and fteady experience, that
they CANNOT " want to be taught;" but
that their judgment, founded upon the beft
bafis, *manual art,* and *ocular infpection,*
OUGHT TO BE much fuperior to any theoretical inftructions that can be obtruded or
enforced. Under that perfuafion, and feeling for thofe *few* who have induftrioufly
rendered themfelves adequate to all the difficulties of the trade, I feel no furprife that
fuch fpirited expoftulations fhould be made,
as muft frequently happen in reply to many
pedantic

pedantic confequential pretenders, who by their *futile remarks* and *ignorant inftruction,* excite the jealous irritability of men, who, confcious of their own ability and integrity, poffefs (like Hotfpur) too much innate fpirit and perfonal courage to be perpetually peftered by " a popping jay."

It has been before obferved, that many horfes have undergone various operations for *fuppofed lameneffes* in different parts, when TIME, and the lucky interpofition of a judicious opinion, have difcovered the caufe to be (where it is too feldom accurately fearched for) in the foot. Lamenefs of this defcription proceeds in general from fome one or other of the following caufes; the nail holes for the faftening of the fhoe to the foot being inferted too far from the outer edge, in the web of the fhoe, and confequently, when *tight clinched,* bearing too hard upon the flefhy edge of the inner fole, conftitutes a preternatural compreffion upon the internal parts and confequent impediment to eafe or action.

Another caufe exceedingly common, (when the

the horfe is faid to be pricked in fhoeing) is the oblique direction of a nail, which taking an improper and inverted courfe, either per-forates, or in its progrefs preffes upon the inner fole, puncturing fome of the foft parts, thereby producing certain lamenefs; which not immediately difcovered, tends to inflammation, that too often terminates in a remote formation of matter conftituting a cafe of the moft ferious confequence.

A third caufe is the inconfiftent method of forming the web of the fhoe too wide for the foot of the horfe, and raifing it fo much, or hollowing it out all round *the inner edge,* as to give it a palpable *convexity* when fixed to the hoof. By this convexity round the inner edge of the web, the fupport be-comes unnaturally partial, and even in the conftant weight of the horfe only (without recurring to action) conftitutes an oppofition to its original purport; for the invariable preffure upon the curved part of the fhoe only, muft raife in the furrounding parts fuch a proportional counteraction, that the harder the horfe bears *in action* upon a hard furface, the more muft every motion tend to force

the

the very nails from their hold, but that the clinches prevent their being withdrawn: In this ftate the horfe, though not abfolutely lame, limps in perpetual uneafinefs, till the clinches of the nails are fo relaxed as to bring the centre nearly to a level with the reft of the foot, where it frequently forms an additional caufe to the original ill, by coming into clofe contact with the fole, which *preffing upon* with any degree of feverity, occafions a flight lamenefs that becomes immediately perceptible.

Another very common caufe of lamenefs with horfes of this defcription originates in the fhoes being formed *too fhort* and *narrow* at the heel, by which means, in lefs than a week's conftant wear, the hoof (or " *cruft*," as fome writers have termed it for the fake of refinement) being alfo *narrow*, the heels of the fhoes make gradual impreffion and conftitute a palpable indentation upon the edge of the fole, directly over its articulation with the hoof, producing to a certainty, if perfevered in, the foundation of *corns*, or a temporary lamenefs, that is generally removed by removing the fhoe.

A few

A few additional bad effects, but of inferior confequence, refulting from injudicious
fhoeing, may be concifely ranged under the
heads of raifing the *fhoes too high in the heels*
without due difcrimination, throwing the fetlock joint into a diftortive pofition ; *corns ill
treated* or *horfes ill fhod,* to occafion the imperfection of *cutting* either before or behind,
an evil arifing much more from want of profeffional accuracy in the operator, than any
abortive effort in the procefs of NATURE.
Thefe are, however, mere fuperficial inconveniencies, to be remedied by fuch attention
and circumfpection as no one friend to the animal we treat of will ever refufe to beftow.

Rules for the prevention or cure of thefe,
are luckily calculated by their brevity for
communication or retention. The heels of
horfes fhould never be artificially raifed only
in exact proportion to the ftate of their feet,
the feafon of the year, and their manner of
going, not without fome additional reference
to the road or country they generally travel ;
all which, every SMITH of the leaft eminence fhould perfectly underftand from *practical experience,* without a long table of conditional

ditional inftructions to fix a criterion, which muft, after all the fpeculative matter or experimental knowledge that can be introduced, be regulated by the exercife of his own profeffional penetration, or the perfonal superintendance of thofe, whofe inftructions it muft be his intereft to obey.

Corns, in general occafioned much more by the unobferved ftricture of the *shoe* (as before defcribed) than any defect in nature, are not fufficiently attended to in their earlieft ftate for fpeedy obliteration; but permitted to acquire by time and continuance of the caufe, a rigid callofity before the leaft attempt is made for extirpation; during which inattention they become fo inflexibly firm in their bafis, that they are not eafily to be eradicated, though great care and perfeverance will greatly affift their mitigation if not entirely eftablish their cure.

The beft and moft confiftent method is to reduce it with the drawing knife, as much as the extent of the corn and the depth of the fole will admit, obferving not to exceed the bounds of difcretion in penetrating the

6   horny

horny fole *too deeply*, rendering by a ftep
of imprudence, the remedy worfe than the
difeafe. When it is thus reduced as much
as the ftate of the corn and the texture of the
foot will juftify, let the entire deftruction of
it be attempted by the occafional application
of a few drops of *oil of vitriol* over its whole
furface; or its rapidity of growth reftrained
by the affiftance of GOULARD's *extract of
faturn, traumatic* (commonly called Friar's)
balfam, camphorated fpirits of wine, or tinc-
ture of myrrh.

This being performed, if the vacuum is
large or *deep* from whence the fubftance has
been extracted, and the operator has been
under the neceffity of nearly perforating the
outer fole, fo as to be productive of additional
tendernefs to the original caufe of complaint;
care muft be taken to prevent the infinuation of extraneous fubftances of different kinds,
as *ftones, gravel, dirt*, or fuch other articles as may very much irritate and injure
the part. This is beft effected by plugging
up the cavity with a pledget of *tow*, firft
hardening the furface well with one of the
before-mentioned fpirituous applications; remembering not to infert the tow too clofely to
                                        deftroy

deftroy its elaftic property, forming a hardnefs from its abundance, that may painfully prefs upon the tender part it is defigned to defend.

It has long been an eftablifhed practice after drawing *a corn*; an injury fuftained in any part of the *hoof*, caufing a partial defect or a difeafed ftate of the *frog*, as inveterate *thrufh*, &c. to protect the part with a *bar fhoe* formed and adapted to fuch purpofe : This is certainly a conditional fecurity, but there is ftill the fpace between the *foot* and the *fhoe* to receive and retain any fubftance, that may become injurious by its lodgment and painful preffure as before-mentioned. To prevent the poffibility of which, I fhould always recommend (in cafes that require it) the infinuation of a fufficient quantity of tow to fill up the interftice ; and that its retention there might be rendered a matter of greater certainty, it fhould be well impregnated with a portion of *diachylon with the gums*, firft melted over the fire ; this will not only fill up the opening with neatnefs (*properly managed*) but form a *bolfter of eafe* to the part, and exclude to a certainty the admiffion of articles we have juft defcribed.

The

The *cutting* of horfes is in general attributed to fome impropriety in the mode of
forming or fetting the fhoe; though this is by
no means to be confidered the *invariable* caufe,
for fuch inconvenience is fometimes produced
by very different means. Horfes, for inftance,
frequently injure themfelves when in too long
and repeated journies they become *leg weary,*
and though of great fpirit and bottom, compulfively fubmit to the power of exhaufted
nature; when hardly able to get one foot before the other, it can create no furprife that
they feel it impoffible to proceed in equal direction, but move their limbs in the moft irregular manner, *warping* and *twifting,* as if
their falling muft prove inevitable at every
fucceffive motion. In fuch ftate of bodily
debilitation, injuries of this kind are undoubtedly fuftained, and too often by the inadvertency or inexperience of the rider or
driver, fuppofed to arife from fome imperfection in the operation of fhoeing, which in
this inftance is no way concerned.

It is not fo in others, where the fhoe being formed too wide for the *hoof,* or with a
projecting fweep at the *heel,* (particularly in
horfes,

horfes, who from an irregular fhape of the foot, called *turning out the toe*, are addicted to a kind of curve in action againft the fetlock joint of the other leg) the evil is conftituted to a certainty; but when it arifes from thefe caufes, it is always to be removed or greatly mitigated by the judicious interpofition of the SMITH, whofe particular province it is to difcover and remedy the defect.

Another caufe of this inconvenience very frequently proceeds from what I have ever confidered a palpable abfurdity in the fyftem of fhoeing, and anxioufly wifh it to undergo a general improvement: This is the *inconfiftent, ridiculous,* and I may almoft venture to add *invincible* folly of forming a *groove* in the web of the fhoe, neither large enough nor deep enough to admit the head of the nail, for the entire reception of which the plan was originally formed; though feldom or ever made fufficiently wide to complete the purport of its firft intention.

The difadvantages arifing from this want (or proftitution) of judgment in execution, is not more the irregular furface of the foot, upon a *hard road* or *pavement*, throwing it unavoidably into a variety of unnatural pofitions by the heads of fome nails being ridiculoufly high or projecting from the fhoe, and others as much below them, than the certainty of all the clinches being raifed in a very few days ufe by the weight and action of the horfe, which on the infide of each foot conftitute the evil to a degree of feverity with horfes that go clofe, particularly if permitted to remain long in fuch ftate unattended to.   Upon expoftulation, you are told, " this is a matter of no inconvenience, that they will foon be worn down and become equal."   If fuch affertion was to be admitted without oppofition refpecting the irregularity of the furface, and diftortive pofitions of the foot, it by no means affects the certainty of rendering the clinches not only evidently injurious in the degree before recited, but of little utility (after a few days wear) in fecuring the fhoe in the fituation it was originally placed.

This is a circumftance fo exceedingly clear, that every rational obferver, poffeffing a defire

to

to promote general improvement, will coincide with me in opinion, and affift the recommendation by the force of example; in having the groove in the web of the fhoe, for the reception of the nails, formed fufficiently wide and deep to admit the heads nearly or quite equal with the flat furface of the fhoe, by which effectual infertion the fhoe firmly retains its fituation, and the nails their clinches, till a repetition of the operation becomes neceffary.

There are (as I have before hinted an intention of explaining) fome general rules to be remembered, as invariably applicable to all kinds of feet without exception. The fhoe fhould be uniformly fupported by the *hoof only*, entirely round the foot, and brought fo regularly into contact, that it fhould not prefs more upon one part than another; it fhould alfo be formed with a concave inner furface, to keep it perfectly clear of the *fole*, that the point of the picker may occafionally pafs under the inner part of the web, to free it from every extraneous or injurious fubftance. The fhoe fhould not be made too wide in the web, or too weighty in metal,

for

for the fize or purpofe of the horfe ; if fo,
the infertion of the nails become unavoidably
neceffary nearer the edge of the flefhy, or
inner fole, and the compreffion upon the internal parts proportionally greater, in the additional hold required, to prevent the inner
edge of the web from finking directly, *by
conftant preffure*, upon the centre of the outer
fole, conftituting certain uneafinefs in action,
if not perceptible lamenefs.   The heel of the
fhoe fhould always rather exceed the termination of the hoof behind, and be formed
fomething *wider* than the heel itfelf; not
only to conftitute a firm bafis of fupport for
the frame, and prevent the *indentation* before
defcribed, but to afford room for the requifite
growth and expanfion of the heel, if a well
formed found foot is at all the object of attention.

The hoofs of horfes fhould never be fuffered to grow *too long at the toe*, for exclufive of its foon conftituting a flat, weak,
narrow foot, it is not uncommonly productive
of *ftumbling* and *tumbling*, to the no great
entertainment, but certain danger of the
rider ; and this frequent error in the prefent

4   practice

practice of fhoeing is the more extraordinary, as the very form, length, and texture of the hoof, will always afford fufficient information in how great a degree it will bear reduction, with the additional confideration, in point of effect, that fhortening *the toe* will always proportionally *widen*, and give ftrength to the *heel*.

Horfes faid to be " flefhy footed," are thofe whofe inner and outer fole are found to be too large in proportion to the fubftance of the hoof that furrounds them; or, in other words, (to render it clear as poffible) whofe hoof is too thin at the lower edge or bottom, for the fize of the whole. This may be productive of inconvenience, and requires a nicer difcrimination in the mode of forming the groove in the web, as well as in fixing the fhoe; for the fpace upon which it muft be unavoidably fixed (without an alternative) is fo exceedingly narrow, that the greateft care and attention is abfolutely neceffary to bring the nails fo near the edge of the hoof, as to avoid every probable chance of injury by too great a ftricture upon the component parts;

N 3

a matter

a matter that has been already more than once concifely recommended to *practical* circumfpection.

That fuch hazard may be the better avoided, it will be found an infurance of fafety; to advance the *front nails* nearer to the extremity of the TOE, where the feat of infertion is much *wider*, and bring the *hinder nails* farther from the points of the HEEL, where it is not only directly the reverfe, but fometimes too narrow to admit of the infertion without danger. And in all cafes where horfes are remarkably full and flefh footed, with a heel exccedingly narrow, it is certainly the fafeft method to let them be fhod with the nails entirely round the front of the foot, omitting their infertion in a proportional degree behind.

LA FOSSE, echoed by BARTLET, condemns the cuftom of turning up the fhoe *at the heels*, upon the before-mentioned objection of its " removing the frog to a greater diftance from the ground, by which the tendon will be inevitably ruptured;" but could they now become fpectators of the hundreds

hundreds of post horses constantly running the roads with BAR SHOES, that totally preclude the *possibility* of the *frogs touching the ground*, to support such elasticity, they might be convinced what little respect such assertion must be held in, under a demonstration exceeding all contradiction. Nor is this retrospective remark brought forward upon any other motive, than to justify the great consistency and safety of judiciously raising the heels of the shoes, to defend frogs that have been bruised, or are naturally defective, and heels that are flat and narrow; as well as to insure the safety of the rider, and prevent the slipping of horses, which must otherways become inevitable in rainy seasons upon chalky roads or hilly countries.

Adverting once more to their promulgation upon "the inconsistency of ever paring the sole or frog," I must avail myself of the present opening to make one addition to my former observations upon that part of the subject; recommending it to the attention of every breeder, to make occasional inspections of the feet even *when yearlings,* and in their progressive gradations, to prevent their

their acquiring an ill conformation : By a want of proper correction they will very frequently be found fpreading to a long flat thin foot, which left to time, will become irrecoverably weak ; on the contrary, proportionally pared at the *battom*, fhortened at the *toe*, and rounded with the rafp, will conftitute the very kind of foot in fhape and firmnefs of all others the moft defirable.

Before we entirely difmifs this fubject, a few remarks upon the management of the feet in *ftabled horfes*, cannot be confidered inapplicable to our prefent purpofe of general utility. Firft, it fhould be remembered, an equal inconvenience arifes from having horfes unneceffarily fhod *too often*, or the ceremony poftponed *too long* ; the former, by its frequency, batters and breaks the hoof (particularly if of the brittle kind) to a perceptible degree of injury ; the latter promotes an aukward growth of the foot, an indentation of the fhoe upon the fole, or inner edge of the hoof, and a probable deftruction of the frog.

Various opinions may have been fupported upon the propriety of ftopping and oiling the

the feet; but as it is not my prefent purpofe to animadvert upon the diffufe remarks
of others, I fhall confine myfelf to practical obfervations of my own. The falutary
effects of plentifully oiling, and nightly
ftopping, the fubftantial, firm, black and
white brittle hoofs, defcribed in a former
page, are too firmly eftablifhed by long and
attentive experience, to render oppofition
(from any authority whatever) worthy a
momentary confideration or condefcending
reply.

A comparative ftate of the hoof that is
carefully managed in this way, with one in
its ftate of nature, (more particularly in the
hot and dry months of fummer) will evidently befpeak the advantage and neatnefs of
fuch care and attention. In one, the hoof
is always in a ftate of pliable uniformity;
in the other, a harfh, conftant and irregular
fcaling of the fole, an almoft inflexible rigidity of the hoof in fhoeing, and moft frequently very large and dangerous cracks that
feparate the *fole* from the *frog* on both fides;
leaving ample room *on either* for the infinuation of fand, gravel, or other injurious articles

ticles that may by their retention reach the coronary articulation, conftituting irreparable lamenefs too frequently attributed to every caufe but the right.

Having gone through fuch chain of inveftigation, and courfe of inftruction, upon the fubject of fhoeing, and its effects, as I conceive to be at all calculated to aflift the general judgment of thofe whofe equeftrian purfuits render fuch knowledge an object of importance; I fhall proceed to that kind of communication, as I flatter myfelf will be equally acceptable to thofe who do me the honour of perufal and attention, whether for amufement, information, literary difquifition, or to render the influence of example, more preferable to precept, by a contribution of their perfonal affiftance to the promotion of general improvement.

STABLING

STABLING

Will prove a chapter more immediately appertaining to the proprietors of extenfive receptacles in the metropolis, as well as other large cities, and thofe interefted in their effects; than at all applicable to the prefent improved ftate of gentlemen's ftables in every part of the kingdom, where the mode of management is approaching too near a degree of perfection to admit the aid of inftruction, from either the pen of theoretic information, or practical experience. As it will, however, be unavoidably neceffary to introduce under this head, fuch occafional remarks or ufeful obfervations as cannot with propriety appear under any other, hints may perhaps be difcovered, in which every reader may feel himfelf *in fome degree* individually concerned.

The very inferior ftate of action and appearance, fo vifibly predominant in horfes of frequent ufe, from the large public livery ftables, when put into competition with

7   hunters

hunters or hacks, enjoying the advantage of regular *food, dreſſing, air,* and *exerciſe,* will conſtitute all the apology I think it neceſſary to introduce, for any degree of freedom I may be inclined to offer, in drawing a compariſon very little obſervable by METROPOLITAN HEROES ON HORSEBACK, but univerſally known to the diſcriminating eye of every experienced ſportſman in the kingdom.

Such inferiority ariſes from an accumulation of cauſes, very little conſidered or enquired into by the owners, or riders, who philoſophically define and experimentally demonſtrate, the horſe to be an animal of general utility, and appropriate him to all their different purpoſes accordingly; with as little attention to his *colour, perfeƈtions,* or *defeƈts,* as a tradeſman of Mancheſter, who having ſome few years ſince occaſion to attend the aſſizes at Lancaſter, hired *a grey gelding* for the purpoſe, but unluckily returned with *a bay mare,* and obſtinately perſiſted (in oppoſition to every witneſs and expoſtulation) that he had brought back *the very horſe* and equipments with which he had

had ftarted, in obedience to the legal in-junction he had received. Of thefe equeftrian Quixotes, nature has been fo exceedingly liberal, that we find numbers, who, when their fteed is brought out of the ftable, whether in *high* or *low* condition, *fee or not fee, fwelled legs, cracked heels, fhoes or no fhoes,* his carcafe expanded to its *utmoft extent,* or contracted to a degree of *unprecedented po-verty;* mount him with equal unconcern, and go through their journey, long or fhort, as prompted by neceffity or inclination, without a fingle reflection upon the wants or weakneffes of the animal, unluckily def-tined to receive the honor of fo *humane* an appendage.

In fuch unaccountable ftate of negligence ftands many a valuable horfe furrounded with an accumulation of ills and hourly promotion of mifery from one week's end to another, and never enjoys the favour (if I may fo term it) of his mafter's prefence but of a *Sunday morning;* when making the expeditious tour of *Richmond, Hampton Court, Windfor,* or fome other of the fafhionable excurfions, he is configned to his ufual hebdomadal *dark*
abode

abode of inactivity, to enjoy a profufion of *hay, water, and eafe ;* but, in conformity with the idea of Major O'Flaherty, " a plentiful fcarcity of every thing elfe."

It is impoffible for any man living, who has made thefe creatures, *their wants, gratifications, perfections,* and *attachments,* the object of his contemplation, not to feel the greateft mortification when chance or choice brings him to a furvey of the ftables in London, with all their horrid inconveniences. To thofe totally unacquainted with the fuperior and fyftematic management of ftables in general, it may all bear the appearance of PROPRIETY, confequently paves no way for the corroding reflections of vexation and difappointment; but to the experienced and attentive obferver, whofe fenfations move in direct unifon with the feelings of the animal he beftrides, and the accommodation of whofe horfe is held in equal eftimation and retention with his own, they excite the joint emotions of pity and furprife.

Horfes in general, produced from ftables of this defcription, all bear the appearance of

temporary

temporary invalids or confirmed valetudi-
narians; from living or rather exifting in a
fcene of almoft total darknefs, they approach
the light with reluctance, and every new
object with additional apprehenfion. They
walk, or rather totter out of the ftable in a
ftate of debilitation and ftiffnefs of the extremities, as if threatened with univerfal
lamenefs. The legs are fwelled from the
knèes and hocks downwards, to the utmoft
expanfion of the integument; which with
the dry and contracted ftate of the *narrow
heeled hoof*, bears no ill affinity to the over-
loaded fhoe of AN OPULENT ALDERMAN,
when emerging from the excruciating admonitions of a gouty monitor. Upon more accurate infpection, we find the lift of happy effects
ftill increafed with thofe ufual concomitants,
inveterate *cracks, running thrufh*, very frequently accompanied by a hufky fhort cough,
or afthmatic difficulty of refpiration, in gradual
progreffion to a broken wind; and the long
lift of inferior *et ceteras*, that conftitute the
invariable advantages of ftable difcipline, directly contrary to every eftablifhed rule that
can be laid down for the promotion of EASE,
HEALTH, and INVIGORATION.

In

In confirmation of which, without a tedious animadversion upon so long a series of inconsistencies, let us advert concisely to the causes of such ill effects as we have ventured to enumerate. The disadvantages arising from horses standing in perpetual darkness, or with a very faint and glimmering light, must be too palpably clear to require much elucidation; for in such state, with the full and increased power of *hearing*, they are incessantly on the watch to discover, what so constantly affects *one sense*, without the expected gratification of *the other*. To this eternal disappointment may be attributed the alternate stare and twinkling of the eye-lids, so common to every description of horses that stand in the most remote part of dark stables, at each time of being brought forward to face the light; as well as the additional observation, that being accustomed to see things but imperfectly in the stable, when brought into action upon the road, they are so much affected by the change, that they become habitually addicted to *stop* or *start* at every strange or sudden object that approaches. A certain danger also attends, when hurried by a careless or drunken ostler, from the external

ternal glare of light to the extreme of total darknefs ; for in fuch hafty tranfition, blows are frequently fuftained againft the racks, ftalls, or intervening partitions, that fome-times terminate in the lofs of *an eye,* with no other caufe affigned for its original appear-ance than the *fluctuation of humours,* which the fuffering fubject immediately undergoes repeated confultations and a long courfe of medicines to eradicate.

The ftiffnefs of the joints, the fwelling of the legs, the feverity of the cracks, the frequency of the thrufh, the contraction of the hoofs, and the difficulty of refpiration, are all fo evidently the refulting effects of deftructive fituation and erroneous manage-ment, that to the fporting world alone, lite-rary definition would be deemed fuperfluous ; but to that infinity of JUVENILE EQUES-TRIANS, who are " daily rifing to our view," and wonder " why their horfes, that they keep *at fo much expence,* are unlike moft others they meet in their rural excur-fions," fuch explanation becomes matter of indifpenfible neceffity.

To the want of general cleanliness, pure
air, and regular exercise, may be juftly attributed all the ills we have juft recited; and
that fuch affertion may lay impartial claim
to proper weight in the fcale of reflection,
let it be firft remembered, that horfes in
the fituation I allude to, are conftantly living in certain degrees of heat, not only beyond the ftate required by nature, but very
far exceeding even the ftable temperature of
horfes in regular training for the turf.

That this may be the better underftood by
thofe whofe fituations in life have precluded
the chance of fuch infpection, and that great
body of readers in various and diftant parts
of the kingdom, who *never have*, and perhaps *never may*, make a furvey of public
ftables in the metropolis; I think it neceffary to introduce an exact reprefentation of
fyftematic inconfiftency, perfectly exculpated
from even the flighteft fufpicion of exaggeration.   As I have repeatedly obferved, and
it is univerfally admitted, there is no rule
without fome exception; fo the following
defcription may have *fome* but VERY FEW
to boaft of.

Upon

Upon entering the major part, (particularly if the door has been a few minutes
clofed and is open for your admiffion) the
olfactory and optic nerves are inftantaneoufly affailed with the volatile effluvia of
dung and *urine*, equal to the exhalation from
a ftock bottle of hartfhorn at the fhop of
any Chemift in the neighbourhood. Here
you find from ten or twelve to twenty
horfes, ftanding as hot, and every crevice
of the ftable as clofely ftopped, as if the
very external air was infectious, and its admiffion muft inevitably propagate a contagion. Naturally inquifitive to difcover what
irritating caufe has laid fuch hold of your
moft prominent feature, you obferve each
horfe ftanding upon an enormous load of
litter, that by occafional additions (without a regular and daily removal from the
bottom) has acquired both the fubftance and
property of a moderate *hot-bed*.

Thus furrounded with the vapours conftantly arifing from an accumulation of the
moft powerful volatile falts, ftand thefe poor
animals a kind of patient facrifice to ignorance
and indifcretion; and that the meafure of

O 2 misery

misery may be rendered perfect by every additional contribution of folly, each horse is absolutely loaded with a profusion of body cloths, but perhaps more to gratify the oftentation or display the opulence of the owner, than any intentional utility to the horse. The sheet, quarter piece, breast cloth, body roller, and perhaps *the hood*, are all brought forward to give proof of persevering attention and unremitting industry. In this state such horses are found upon critical examination, to be in an almost perpetual languid perspiration; so debilitated, depressed, and inactive, for want of pure air and regular exercise, that they appear dull, heavy, and inattentive, as if conscious of their imprisonment and bodily persecution.

The effect of this mode of treatment soon becomes perceptible to the judicious eye of observation; the carcase is seen unnaturally full and overloaded, for want of those gradual evacuations promoted by gentle motion; the legs swell, becoming stiff and tumefied, till nature, in her utmost efforts for extravasation, terminates in either *cracks, scratches, grease,* or some one of the many

disorders

disorders arising from an impurity, viscidity, or acrimony in the blood. The hoofs by being almost invariably fixed to the constant heat of the accumulating dung before described, acquires a degree of contraction indicating hoof-bound lameness. The eyes frequently give proof of habitual weakness, in a watery discharge from the continual irritation of the volatile effluvia, the dilatation and contraction of the eye in search of light, the heat of the body, &c. all tending to constitute a frame directly opposite in health, vigour, and appearance, to those whose *condition* is regulated by a very different system of stabularian management.

The evils arising from this mistaken treatment are only yet enumerated in part, being those that evidently appear upon a superficial survey of the stables and their contents; others become discernible upon being brought into action. They are certainly less enabled to encounter fatigue than any horses in the kingdom; from so constant an existence in the *absolute fumes of a hot-bath*, they never can be exposed to the external air in a *cold*, *wet*, or *winter* season, without danger to

O 3 every

every part of the frame. By fuch contract they are inftantly liable to a fudden collapfion of the porous fyftem, which locking up the perfpirative matter, fo violently propelled to the furface, throws it back upon the circulation with redoubled force; where nature being too much overloaded to admit its abforption, it becomes immediately fixed upon the EYES or LUNGS, laying a very fubftantial foundation of difeafe and difquietude.

If fuch horfe is put into ftrong exercife, he foon proves himfelf inadequate to either a long, or an expeditious journey; for whether the body is overburthened with weak and flatulent food and water at fetting out, jaded with early fatigue, to which he has not been accuftomed, or debilitated with the ftable difcipline we have fo minutely defcribed, the effect is nearly the fame. If his journey is of any duration, or his exertions of any great magnitude, it is no uncommon thing to find he has fallen *fick, lame,* or *tired* upon the road; and under the worft of curfes, *a bad character,* is frequently fold to the firft bidder; under whofe

3   fyftematic

fyftematic care and rational mode of management, a few months perhaps makes him
one of the beft and moft valuable horfes
in the kingdom.

This is a circumftance that happens fo
very conftantly in the equeftrian fluctuation
of fortune, and the affertion fo repeatedly
juftified by ocular demonftration and practical experience, that I ftand not in the
leaft fear of a contrariety of opinions upon
fo confpicuous a part of the fubject.

The ill effects of the ftable treatment
we have hitherto defcribed, would be ftill
more injurious did *high feeding* conftitute a
part of the fyftem we prefume to condemn ;
but a *fuper-abundance* of food is what I by
no means place to the *inconfiftency* of the
account. Prudence (divefted of *felf-intereft*)
powerfully prompts the parties concerned,
to perceive the *abfurdity* of *over-feeding*
horfes whofe ftate fo little requires it. Stable keepers are not fo deftitute of PENE-
TRATION, as to be taught by me, the *folly*
of feeding horfes that " *don't work.*" OATS
are not only unneceffary but *fuperfluous* ; hay

in

in *small quantities* will support nature suffi-ciently, by a constant mastication of which the appetite will be properly prepared to receive PLENTY OF WATER; an article that is not only of very little expence and trou-ble, but by expanding the frame, and filling the flank, will afford to the *city sportsman* and *Sunday traveller*, sufficient proof that the horse is *amply fed*, and " *well looked after.*"

Having submitted to consideration the representation of FACTS, that neither the interested *can*, or the experienced *will*, at-tempt to deny; I shall (without much hope of effecting a reformation where so great a variety of opinions are concerned) beg permission to offer a few remarks, for the attention of those who are, from the nature of their situations, unavoidably con-nected with stables of this description; leaving the more minute instructions for the management of hunters or road horses, to be collected from the matter that will be hereafter introduced under those heads.

The pernicious properties of *foul air* must be

be too well known, or at leaft too readily comprehended, (by every one to whofe ferious perufal thefe pages will become fubject) to require even the moft fuperficial elucidation; though in fact, entering into its deftructive effects, with all its contingent confequences, would be to *write, quote,* and animadvert a volume upon the fubject; which is in fact of too much fcientific magnitude for prefent difquifition, in a publication that promifes to be generally read, and it is intended fhould be as generally underftood.

Under palpable conviction of the numerous ills that may arife in different ways from air fo very much contaminated, and replete with impurities, I am convinced no one advocate for improvement can rationally object to the adoption of VENTILATORS in all public ftables, where the fituation is inevitably confined; as in London, and other large cities, where they muft unavoidably continue fo without the moft diftant probability of rectification.

The utility, the convenience, the exhilarating

rating rays of " ALL CHEARING LIGHT,"
(that enables us to enjoy fociety, for which
we were formed) is a matter standing in no
need of *tedious* recommendation; it therefore cannot be too forcibly inculcated, or too
cheerfully adopted.

Cleanlinefs is fo indifputably necefiary to
health and invigoration, that it is matter of
furprife how fo palpable a fyftem of filth
could ever be permitted to pervade the
equeftrian receptacles of thofe who would,
no doubt, be exceedingly hurt and offended,
if they were to have the inconfiftencies of
their conduct perfonally demonftrated, and
be compulfively convinced they either *do not
know* or *feem to care* any thing about the
matter.   In fact, there is but one reafon
that can be urged, (and none with fo much
energy as thofe prompted by felf-intereft)
in favour of a practice replete with fo many
difadvantages; this muft be the high price
and difficulty of obtaining ftraw in the metropolis, which in its transformation to
manure becomes fo reduced to a mere no-
thingnefs in value, that the *poffibility* of being

ing cleanly in thofe ftables (we are told) is abfolutely precluded by pecuniary confide-rations. But when the fixed emoluments of the *weekly keep* are taken into the aggre-gate, and it is not the effect of rumination but matter of fact, that many of the horfes *fo kept*, are, from want of exercife and the numerous caufes before affigned, fo very much OFF THEIR APPETITES, as not to confume in a day but *one* or *two* of the *four feeds* of corn that are charged; an extra trufs of ftraw from the loft LIBERALLY EXCHANGED for each bufhel and a half of oats *accidentally* faved in the granary, would certainly prove no violent proftitution of generofity !

E X E R C I S E,

Is a matter of too much importance in the promotion of health and condition to be excluded its place in our prefent arrange-ment ; and fo evidently neceffary to the na-tural fecretions and regular evacuations, that the foundation of every difeafe may be laid

by

by a want of it. Horfes are in their very nature and difpofition fo formed for motion, that they become dull, heavy, and unhealthy without it; of this nothing can afford greater demonftration than the pleafure they difplay in every action, when brought from the dark recefs of a gloomy ftable to the perfect enjoyment of light, air, and exercife. The natural fweetnefs of the external air is fo happily fuperior to the ftagnate impurity of the ftable, that moft horfes inftantly exult in the change, and by a variety of ways convince you of the preference.

Survey a fpirited horfe with the eye of attention, and obferve the aftonifhing difference *before* and *after* his liberation - from the *manger*, to which he is fometimes, under the influence of ftrange mifmanagement, haltered for days together without remiffion. In the ftable you perceive him *dejected, fpiritlefs,* and almoft inanimate, without the leaft feeming courage or activity in his compofition; but when brought into action, he inftantly affumes another appearance, and indicates by bodily exultation and exertion,

ertion, the abfolute falubrity and neceffity of what the inftinctive ftupidity of many can never (from their inexplicable want of com-prehenfion) be brought to underftand. Such inconfiderate obfervers might certainly im-prove their *very fhallow judgment,* by fome trifling attention to the indications of nature in horfes of any tolerable defcription, who all difplay, in different attitudes and by va-rious means, the gratification they enjoy in their diftinct appropriations. In fact, the animated afpect of the whole frame, the live-ly eye, the crefted neck, the tail erect, with the moft fpirited bodily action of neighing, fnorting, and curvetting, all tend to prove the conftitutional utility of exercife in length and manner adapted to the fize, ftrength, make, condition, and purpofe of the horfe.

Perfectly convinced of its indifpenfible neceffity to horfes of all kinds, in propor-tion to the ufes for which they are defigned, and the portion of aliment they receive, I am not unfrequently very highly entertain-ed with the management of many within the extenfive circle of my own acquaint-ance, (and thofe too with inherent pride

2   fufficient

sufficient to assume the character of sportf-
men) who are in constant possession of good
and valuable horses, perpetually *buying, fell-
ing,* and *exchanging* ; but never for years together, have one in their stables *three months,*
without swelled legs, cracked heels, grease,
bad eyes, broken knees, or some of the many
ills that constitute a stable of infirmities ; all
which they very PHILOSOPHICALLY and
erroneously attribute to *ill luck,* that I most
justly and impartially place to the account of
inadvertent masters, and much more indolent
servants.

The advantages arising from an unremitting perseverance in the regularity of
daily exercise, (both in respect to time and
continuance) cannot be so clearly known
and perfectly understood, but to those who
have attended minutely to the good effects
of its practice, or the ills that become
constantly perceptible from its omission.
This *is* undoubtedly the more extraordinary, when it is recollected there is no one
part of the animal œconomy more admirably adapted to the plainest comprehension,
than the system of repletion and evacuation ;

which

which may (avoiding technical defcription
and profeffional minutiæ) be concifely explained and clearly underftood, as matter
neceffarily introductory to what we proceed
to inculcate, upon the palpable confiftency
of conftant and moderate exercife for the
eftablifhment of health and promotion of
condition.

I believe it has been before faid, in either this or the former volume, that the
ALIMENT, after fufficient maftication in
the act of chewing, is paffed to the ftomach,
where it undergoes regular fermentation (in
general termed digeftion) producing a certain quantum of *chyle*, in proportion to the
nutritive property of the aliment fo retained :
This chyle, in its procefs of nature; (which
has been before accurately explained) becomes
wonderfully fubfervient to all the purpofes of
life and fupport in its general contribution to
the fource of circulation, and the various fecretions; while the groffer parts (from which
the nutritious property is extracted in their
progrefs through the ftomach and inteftinal
canal) are thrown off from the body by excrementitious evacuations.

This

This is a concise abstract of nature's operation; as necessary to constitute sufficient information to comprehend our present purpose of explicit animadversion upon the great advantage of bodily motion, so far as it shall appear conducive to the preservation of health.   Enough is consequently advanced to gratify every competent idea; and afford ample conviction, that should the body be permitted to receive, and continue to accumulate in the frame, more ALIMENT than can be absorbed into the circulation, and carried off by the different emunctories in *a certain portion of time*; over repletion, disquietude, and ultimately DISEASE, acute or chronic, must be the inevitable consequence.

The system and effect are too palpably clear to be at all mistaken in even a theoretic survey of the process; for when the blood vessels become over-loaded with an accumulated retention of perspirable matter, and the stomach and intestines preternaturally extended by indurated excrement (all which should be occasionally carried off by exercise) indisposition must arise in a greater

or

or lefs degree, fo foon as the repletion produces oppreffion, that the ftruggling efforts
of nature are unable to fubdue.

Thefe unembellifhed facts are too plain
and ftriking to require much time from the
WRITER, or patience from the READER,
for farther inveftigation or comprehenfion ; concluding, therefore, this part of
the *animal mechanifm* is perfectly underftood, I fhall proceed to an explanation
of the *active caufes* of fuch diforders as
originate in impurities of the blood, occafioned by want of motion and confequent
evacuation.

It is therefore neceffary we take a furvey
of a horfe brought from the ftable in a
ftate of plenitude after temporary inactivity,
when we find the body too full and over-
loaded to make his firft efforts with any
degree of eafe or pleafure ; every one not
totally abforbed in a ftate of ftupefaction or
natural illiteracy, muft have obferved the
unremitting *attempts* and *ftrainings* of the
animal to throw off the fuperfluous burthen
by repeated evacuations fo foon as brought

into action. If at all hurried before the carcafe is in fome degree relieved from its accumulated contents, you perceive a wheezing or difficulty of refpiration, occafioned by the preffure of the ftomach thus loaded, upon the lobes of the lungs, reftraining them in their natural elafticity for the purpofes of expanfion and contraction.

In this ftate alfo, if his pace is extended beyond a walk, you find him break into a more violent perfpiration than a horfe in proper condition and regular exercife would difplay in a long journey, continued at the fame rate, without intermiffion. Thefe are all indications of nature not to be miftaken or denied, by thofe at all connected or converfant with the fubject before us, and fufficiently demonftrate the refulting effects of continuing to over-load the fyftem with a greater quantity of food than there is proportional exercife to carry off.

PERSPIRATION (that is the gradual emiffion phyfically termed infenfible, as not being profufe to perception) will, in even *gentle exercife*, take from the fuperflux of

the

the BLOOD, what the neceffary evacuations of *dung* and *urine* take from the accumulated contents of the INTESTINES; which fuffered to remain in an abundant and preternatural proportion, muft, by its compulfive retention, acquire a degree of putrid or acrimonious morbidity inevitably producing difeafe. Thefe morbid attacks act differently upon different fubjects, according to their ftate or tendency, at the time of the blood or body's affuming a corrupt or infectious influence; difplaying itfelf in fuch way as is moft applicable to the conftitutional predominance of difeafe in the horfe previous to the leaft trait of difcovery.

I fhall, in compliance with my promife in the introductory part of this work, forbear to lead the reader farther into a tedious train of remote medical refearches, but refer him to the different difquifitions of the former volume for any gratification he may wifh to obtain; letting it fuffice to obferve, that from fuch original caufe may arife the various diftreffing difquietudes fo repeatedly enumerated, as fwelled legs, cracked

P 2   heels,

heels, greafe, afthmatic cough, fret, ftrangury, farcy, fever, convulfions, or in fact any of the numerous difeafes to which horfes are fo conftantly liable.

Thefe caufes of the various difeafes, fo perfectly clear not only to every fcientific inveftigator but every rational obferver, are what have for time immemorial, in the fta-bularian dialect, paffed under the *undefined* denomination of HUMOURS, with the numerous tribe of equeftrian dependents, from the firft ftud groom of the firft fporting nobleman, to the moft illiterate ftable boy in the kingdom; without a fingle profef-fional exertion of refpectability, to wipe away the abftrufe and ignorant fubterfuge of attributing the generality of diforders to the effect of *humours*, without any per-fpicuous attempt to explain in their different publications, what they have univer-fally taken the liberty to condemn.

I am exceedingly forry to fay (and fay it I do, not from any intentional oppofition or difrefpect to the writers) that the more I compare former literary opinions with experimental

perimental practice, the less reason I find to be satisfied with what they ventured to promulgate; particularly upon the subject of *humours*, which in all my enquiries and minute investigations, I could never find systematically explained, at least to encounter the eye of professional inspection.

BRACKEN, who for years was considered a prodigy of VETERINARIAN instruction, after condemning the farriers frequent use and the convenient subterfuge of the word, makes many efforts to go through an elaborate explanation, that, he says, "the ignorance and stupidity of the vulgar are inadequate to;" but very unluckily, after attacking the subject in *nine different ways*, at least in as many different places, he as repeatedly digresses from the point, without ever coming into the *probability* of an explanatory conclusion.

BARTLET, in his usual condescending stile of imitation, (or rather compilation) affords *six pages* of duodecimo, replete with technical abstrusity, collected from the remote allusions and eccentric remarks of his

P 3   learned

learned predeceffor; beginning with a promife of unlimitted explanation, and *almoft immediately* taking leave with the following apology, that " what ought to be underftood by the word HUMOURS, would take up more time than the brevity we have prefcribed ourfelves will admit on."

Taking no more time from the reader than is neceffary to explain what has been already introduced, and to juftify what is to follow, upon the *hacknied fubjeƐt of humours*; I advert to fuch profeffional remarks as have arifen from attentive obfervation, with occafional oblique references to the opinions of thofe who have gone before us, fraught with temporary popularity; having for fuch introduction, no motive but an eager and acknowledged defire to eftablifh the TRUTH, by a proper and incontrovertible criterion of practical inveftigation.

Admitting, therefore, the repletion arifing from a fuperflux of alimentary nutriment, (not carried off by thofe gradual excretions promoted by moderate exercife in *gentle motion*) to conftitute what has fo long paffed
under

under the vague denomination of *humours*, without a fear of being controverted by any refpectable opponent; I fhall proceed to the proper mode of rectification in fuch cafe, and the degree of diftinction to be afcertained when fome of the difeafes before-mentioned proceed from a different caufe.

To effect this, it is firft neceffary to obferve, that when fuch repletion becomes perceptible, and is *immediately* counteracted by regular and daily increafing exercife, it may probably (if the horfe is in no confirmed ftate of foulnefs) be again abforbed into the circulation, and carried off without the affiftance of extra evacuations promoted by medicine. But it fhould be always held in remembrance, that fuch exercife muft be in the firft inftances, not only of great gentlenefs but long duration; ufing no violence or fpeedy exertions, till the body is by gradual perfeverance perfectly unloaded, and the carcafe and extremities have recovered their original form and pliability; when the exercife may be increafed to a greater degree of action, that the fuper-

fluous

fluous and offending matter thus abforbed, may tranfpire by the moft natural effort of perfpiration.

To promote which, with the greater fafety and facility, BLEEDING fhould pre-cede in proportion to *fize*, *ftrength*, and *condition*, that the real ftate of the blood fhould be the more clearly afcertained ; as may be found particularly explained in va-rious parts of the former volume, where it is abfolutely neceffary its predominant ap-pearance fhould undergo critical examina-tion. But in this confcientious recommen-dation, I am unavoidably drawn into ad-ditional remarks upon the opinions of others ; to demonftrate the inconfiftency of *theirs*, as a neceffary prelude to the juftice and eftablifhment of my *own*. And I muft confefs it gives me fome concern, that I am under the neceffity of differing *in a fingle opinion* from authority fo very refpect-able, and judgment fo truly profeffional, as his Majefty's Farrier for Scotland, whofe elegant publications entitle him to univerfal applaufe, for the great pains he has taken to elucidate and improve, a fyftem that has

has for ages remained in an acknowledged
ftate of barbarity and ignorance.

Mr. Clarke, in his " Obfervations on
Blood Letting," fays " It is difficult to fix
any precife ftandard, how we may judge
either of the healthy or morbid ftate of
the blood in horfes when cold." This is
an opinion fo directly oppofite to what
I have frequently advanced upon former
occafions, (with reafons at large for infpecting it in fuch ftate) that my filence
upon the paffage alluded to, would bear fo
much the appearance of pufillanimity or
profeffional ignorance, that I gladly avail
myfelf of the prefent opportunity to fubjoin
a few words in fupport of the opinion formerly maintained ; but with the moft unfullied refpect for a writer of fo much perfpicuity and eminence, whofe abilities I hold in
the greateft eftimation.

It may, as Mr. Clarke feems to think,
" be difficult to fix any *precife ftandard* to
difcover the exact ftate of the blood when
cold ;" but I doubt not his candour, upon due
deliberation, will admit the CERTAINTY
of

of diftinguifhing its property, or predominant tendency, *much better* in that condition, than a ftate of liquidity as juft received from the vein. If that *certainty* is
admitted, (as I flatter myfelf it will not,
upon reflection, be refpectably denied) it
muft undoubtedly prove much more eligible and fatisfactory to obtain profeffional
prognoftics IN PART, than not to acquire
any information *at all*. This being a pofition beyond the power of confutation, it
is only neceffary to add a fingle remark
arifing from daily practice, long experience, and accurate obfervation, upon the
certainty of afcertaining from a minute examination of *the blood when cold*, the proportion of CRASSAMENTUM, SERUM, SIZE,
VISCIDITY, probable inflammation or acrimony it contains; from all which, furely
diagnoftics may be rationally formed to regulate future proceedings; at leaft, fo I conftantly find it in the courfe of my own
practice; and until fuch infpection, by any
deception, fhould convince me of its uncertainty and inutility, I fhall not be readily induced to alter an opinion founded
upon practical conviction; though I muft

acknowledge there is no publication upon thefe fubjects extant, to whofe dictates I fhould more cheerfully become a convert, than the productions of the very author, whofe opinion, *in one inftance,* I am compelled to oppofe.

It is fo perfectly in point to adopt the vulgarifm of " killing two birds with one ftone," that I cannot refift the temptation and prefent opportunity to introduce a few words upon an inconfiftent paffage in BRACKEN, that equally clafhes with an opinion of mine frequently introduced in my former volume, where the operation of BLEEDING, or the *ftate of the blood,* neceffarily became matter of recommendation. In page 111 of his fecond volume, he fays, " the blood becomes vifcid, poor, and difpirited." This paffage is fo ftrangely fequeftered from comprehenfion, fo ridiculoufly replete with paradoxical obfcurity, and fo directly contrary to my own obfervations, founded in practice, and long fince communicated under the fanction of inviolate veracity, that I cannot permit fuch a profufion of profeffional contrarieties to

pafs

pa*s* current upon the public, without ob-
truding a few words to elucidate, or rather
expofe the myftery.

To eftablifh the credit and juftify the
reputation of " The Stable Directory," as
well as to obtain the approbation of thofe
who at no time condemn without infpection, or applaud without reafon ; I have
never advanced *an opinion*, or reported *a
fact*, but what has been founded upon
principles of incontrovertible information
or acknowledged utility. It has been my
invariable ftudy to enlighten, not to perplex ; what has been too much the fyftem
of other writers upon fimilar fubjects, may
be more properly collected from a revifion
of their productions, than the pen of a competitor. But I will venture to affirm, if
any part of my obfervations had contained
fo many abfurd contrarieties, or tedious
and inapplicable digreffions, as the elaborate volumes of BRACKEN ; the *tenth edition* of the former volume, or the title page
of the *fecond*, could never have met the
light, in the prefent enlightened fcene of
equeftrian enquiry and literary improvement.

ment. On the contrary, had I proftituted my judgment or my pen, to fo unfcientific a declaration as the blood's being " *vifcid, poor,* and *difpirited,*" the united force of menftrual criticifm, would have irrevocably doomed ME AND MY OPINIONS to the *loweft region* of oblivion.

How, at the *fame time,* blood can be " VISCID and POOR," or the two words of a direct contrary meaning become fo conveniently fynonimous, I am at a lofs to learn; but perfectly anxious that the profeffional confiftency, the fyftematic uniformity of my affertions, may be arraigned and brought to iffue with opinions fo directly oppofite, I find it unavoidably neceffary, to folicit from every impartial inveftigator, a comparative view of what has been advanced *on either fide* refpecting the blood, when he will be enabled to decide, whofe fyftem approaches neareft to truth, fupported by reafon.

To juftify and corroborate my remarks upon Mr. Clarke's idea of " not difcovering ing the true ftate of the blood when cold," I muft beg to repeat the very words of my

6
opinion

opinion PREVIOUSLY given to the public in the former volume, clafs the third, under the head " FARCY," where will be found the following defcription, neceffarily *again* fubmitted to the difquifition of every enlightened reader.

" In refpect to cure, upon the very earlieft appearance, take away blood in quantity as before defcribed ; and after fo doing, attend minutely to the QUALITY, which circumftances will enable you to form a very decifive judgment, how foon and to what proportion the fubject will bear this evacuation, fhould it again be neceffary ; for according to the extra proportion of the *Craffamentum*, or *Coagulum*, and the fize (or gelatinized fubftance upon the furface) with the difproportion of ferum or watery part, it may be very readily afcertained how much the blood is certainly *above* or *below* the ftandard of mediocrity neceffary for the abfolute PRESERVATION of health."

This is the opinion originally held forth in my firft publication, and with fo firm an adherence to truth, founded upon experience, that

that I never (particularly after so much additional practice and investigation) can conde-
scend to change my opinion, and admit its
uncertainty, in compliment to the unsupported
ipse dixit of any pen whatever; and that I may
stand totally exculpated from the charge of
publishing an opinion so contrary to the respec-
table authority of Mr. Clarke, I must beg to
observe, that my opinion had not only the
priority of his in publication, but had been in
circulation full TWO YEARS before Mr.
Clarke's treatise came into my possession.

We come now to the *judicious* declaration
of BRACKEN, respecting the blood that he
calls " *viscid, poor,* and *dispirited*;" to correct which unaccountable professional slip,
the above quotation will in a certain degree
contribute; particularly when I submit it to
recollection, that in many parts of my former volume (appropriated entirely to medical
researches) I have represented *viscid, sizey*
blood, to be the resulting effect of too much
plenitude arising from alimentary repletion
with a want of proper exercise; while, on
the contrary, I have described too great a
portion of *serum* to constitute an *impover-*
ished

ished blood in being deprived of its due proportion of CRASSAMENTUM, as before recited.

To renew and corroborate which, I muſt be permitted to recommend to the retroſpective attention of thoſe, anxious to diſtinguiſh between the ſpecious deluſion of *theory* and the eſtabliſhment of fact, my obſervations in the ſame claſs, under the article of " MANGE." where it will be found I have defined the poverty of the blood in the following explanatory paſſage.

" For the blood being by this barren contribution robbed of what it was by nature intended to receive, becomes impoveriſhed even to a degree of incredibility (by thoſe unacquainted with the ſyſtem of repletion and circulation) ; it loſes its tenacity and *balſamic adheſive* quality, degenerating to an acrid ſerous vapour, that acquires malignity by its preternatural ſeparation from its original *corrector.*"

Theſe explanations are ſo phyſically correct, ſo perfectly clear, and ſo evidently
adapted

adapted to every comprehenfion, that I am fatisfied to reft the certainty of its procefs, and my own profeffional reputation, upon the arbitrative decifion of any impartial invefti-gator. And that this comparative procefs may be brought to a fpeedy termination, I fhall only beg leave to obferve, if Mr. CLARKE's *hypothefis*, " that no difcovery can be made from the blood when *cold*," is a fact, or the " *vifcid*, *poor*, and *difpirited blood*" of BRACKEN, can be defined one and the fame thing, divefted of paradoxical com-plication, and fuch eccentric opinions are founded *in truth*, and can be fupported by *incontrovertible facts* ; my affertions, however fcientific, however eftablifhed by TIME, and confirmed by EXPERIENCE, muft inevitably fall unfupported to the ground, unworthy the future attention of thofe by whofe approbation and applaufe I have been fo highly honoured.

Having endeavoured to refcue from public prejudice, any hafty decifions that might be made upon fuch clafhing opinions *undefined* ; we return to the operation of bleeding, re-commended previous to the conftant exer-cife, and with that bleeding an accurate exa-mination

mination of the blood WHEN COLD; and this upon the basis of my former opinion again repeated, that should the *craffamentum* (or coagulum) be proportionally greater in quantity to the *ferum* (or watery part) than the *ferum* to the *coagulum*, I should not hesitate a moment to pronounce such horse to be *above himself* in condition, more particularly if the blood had acquired a *vifcid tenacity*, perceptible upon its furface.

When I say above himself in condition, I wish to be underftood, he is in the very ftate we have already defcribed, viz. the whole frame is over-loaded by a fuper-abundance of nutriment, not carried off by exercife; and the impurities thus collected, to have no reference to latent difeafe, but merely the effect of fuch fuperflux fufpended in the conftitution, producing a temporary ftagnation of what I have already defined HUMOURS to be, for want of gradual motion and confequent evacuations. This being the exact ftate of a horfe labouring under plethora and its concomitants from fulnefs only, I should immediately adopt the ufe of a mash each night, compofed of *malt* and *bran*, equal parts, merely to foften the indurated contents of
the

the inteſtines, and promote their more expeditious diſcharge during the gradual exerciſe in the following days; exciting the
veſſels to an increaſed ſecretion of *urine*
by the interpoſition of *two ounces of nitre,*
thoroughly diſſolved in the water of each
morning, when horſes will in general drink
it with a greater degree of avidity. This
plan regularly perſevered in for ſix or eight
days, with daily increaſing exerciſe and good
ſubſtantial dreſſings in the ſtable (more particularly patient rubbing of the legs downwards) may be reaſonably expected to carry
off the repletion, *in part, or all,* according
to the ſtate and condition of the horſe, or the
time of its accumulation.

On the contrary, ſhould the blood in five
or ſix hours after it is taken away, be found to
contain but a ſmall portion of CRASSAMEN-
TUM, in proportion to the much greater of
SERUM; and ſuch coagulum to be of a
florid healthy appearance, I could not doubt
even for a moment but ſuch ſwellings of
the legs, cracks, greaſe, defluxions of the
eyes, (or any other complaints uſually ariſing
from ſuch cauſe) may be the effect of an

Q 2

acrimo-

acrimonious, impoverifhed, and difeafed ftate of the blood; for the due correcting of which, proper remedies may be felected from the former volume of this work, under the different claffes and heads to which they are the moft applicable.

Defluxions of the eyes arifing from whatever caufe, whether the *repletion* already defined, that by its accumulation diftends the finer veffels in proportion as the larger are over-loaded, and in fuch retention acquires tendency to difeafe; from fuch external injuries as *bites* and *blows*; or a relaxed, defective, or paralytic affection of the internal organs, they are all in general denominated HUMOURS *without diftinction*, and phyfically treated accordingly. Hence arifes a very predominant and almoft univerfal error, for want of judicious difcrimination in paying proper attention to the ftate of the blood; the difference and property of which have been fo accurately and repeatedly defcribed, that there is no opening left to admit the plea of ignorance in any one cafe where it is entitled to infpection.

If

If a threatened diforder in the eye is fuppofed to be the effect of repletion and refulting *vifcidity*, fome judgment may be formed from a minute examination of the blood, which will bear refemblance to the ftate accurately explained when the horfe is too much *above himfelf in condition*, and the veffels more or lefs overcharged with impurities.   Exclufive of a fole dependence upon which prognoftic, much information may be collected from external appearance; the eyes are full, heavy, and dull, with an apparent tendency to inflammation in the lids above and below, and exceedingly turbid in the centre; difplaying in fuch ftate a perpetual drowfinefs, his eyes being frequently clofed when ftanding in the ftable undifturbed and feemingly unperceived, but without *the leaft difcharge* tending to difcover the original caufe of complaint.

On the contrary, when arifing from an impoverifhed and acrimonious ftate of the blood, the eyes become upon the firft attack full and inflamed; almoft immediately difcharging a fharp fcalding ferum, that is inceffantly rolling down the cheeks, and in its

Q 3   paffage

paffage (by its conftant heat and irritation) frequently occafions excoriation; the eye gradually contracting and finking in its orbit, in proportion to the length and inveteracy of difeafe. This defluxion is fo very oppofite in caufe and effect, and requires a fyftem of treatment fo very different to the cafe juft defcribed, as arifing from *a vifcidity in the blood*, (conftituting HUMOUR of a diftinct kind) that a nicer judgment is neceffary than generally exerted in fuch difcrimination.

In cafes where one eye only is affected in either of the ways before-defcribed, it may with a great degree of reafon be attributed to *external* injury, and the refulting pain, inflammation, or difcharge, fo far dependent upon the original caufe as to be merely fymptomatic; unlefs from the great irritability and exquifite fenfation of the part, fome of the humours of the eye fhould be fo feverely injured as to occafion its lofs; a circumftance that is too frequently known to happen by an accidental blow, but undoubtedly many more by thofe wilfully aimed and fatally executed.

As

As I have before obferved, one grand error has formerly arifen, and is ftill continued by all the advocates for, and invincible followers of *Ancient Farriery*, to treat " the HUMOURS that have fallen into the eyes" (making ufe of their own language) exactly in the fame way; whether they proceed from any of the caufes juft recited, or the long lift of poffibilities that might be added to the catalogue. It is really in reflection a dreadful confideration, that experience enables me to proclaim fo ferious a fact, and with variety of proofs to eftablifh the certainty, that more horfes are deprived of their eyes and rendered totally blind, by the unbounded ignorance, quackery, and felf-fufficiency of *fome*, with the confidence and affected medical knowledge of *others*, than any bodily difeafe or local defect to which the frame is fubject in the courfe of nature.

It is a matter of no fmall concern to thofe who wifh to fee a rapid improvement in the medical management of this ufeful animal, to find *in cafes of confequence*, upon every enquiry to difcover the caufe and what methods

Q 4 have

have been taken to relieve, all the information must be derived from interrogatories to the *servant*; who is in general possessed of *all the mystery*, and the MASTER (however valuable the horse) is frequently found to know little or nothing at all of the matter. The groom's judgment is in general so perfectly *infallible*, that it would be absolute presumption in his employer, to enquire into the cause of complaint or method of cure; yet upon accurate investigation of these *extensive abilities*, we find very slender cause for the unlimited confidence and implicit opinion of the master. If enquiry is made whether the horse has been bled, and we are answered he has, we are already arrived at the ultimatum of information; for what *quantity* was taken away, or what *quality* it was WHEN COLD, must remain in its former obscurity; one general answer suffices for every question; and with a blush of *conscious stupidity*, we are told, the horse was " *bled on the dunghill.*" By this specimen of enlightened information, every additional suggestion may may be fairly supposed equally *conclusive* and *satisfactory*.

However,

. However, to avoid farther digreſſion in the preſent inſtance, and come to a palpable demonſtration of an aſſertion juſt made ; I ſhall very conciſely introduce from the multiplicity that have occurred, two recent caſes only, as directly applicable to our preſent purpoſe of corroboration ; and it is rather remarkable they ſhould both happen on the ſame day, and within a very ſhort time of this repreſentation going to preſs, the horſes being the property of perſons of the firſt faſhion, and each of them ſent upwards of *twenty miles* for my opinion.

The firſt was a HUNTER of high qualifications and conſiderable eſtimation ; upon accurate examination I found him in the exact ſtate I have deſcribed when labouring under a defluxion of the eyes, (ariſing from a diſeaſed and acrimonious ſtate of the blood) the diſcharge from which, in its long continuance and ſeverity, had " fretted channels in his cheeks ;" the eyes were ſo very much periſhed that they were abſolutely contracted in their orbs, the frame weak and emaciated, diſplaying a ſpectacle with very ſlender and diſcouraging hopes of rectification.

Anxious

Anxious to obtain every poffible information upon fo extraordinary and unpromifing a cafe, I commenced my enquiry with caution, and continued it with precifion, to the attainment of every particular ftep that had been taken for his relief; and doubt not but every reader will be as much furprifed in the perufal, as I muft have been in the recital, when he is informed, that the horfe had been in this gradually encreafing ftate for two months; with the additional mortification to the parties, that every method adopted for his improvement had evidently contributed to his difadvantage.

Every degree of admiration, however naturally excited by the force of this reflection, will as naturally fubfide when the communication of the meffenger and the ftate of the horfe have undergone a little deliberative retrofpection. In the firft inftance, his keep was fo reduced as barely to fubfift nature; he had undergone *five bleedings*, (without the leaft reference to either *quantity* or *quality*) three dofes of ftrong mercurial phyfic, two ounces of nitre a day from the origin of complaint; and *laftly*, to render complete a
fyftem

syftem of inconfiftencies, A ROWEL had been inferted, as if the whole procefs had been intentionally calculated to encreafe the caufe and inveteracy of difeafe. From the ill effects of this cafe (which is critically accurate and authentic) may be derived a leffon of the greateft utility to thofe who, perfectly happy in the vortex of perfonal confidence and felf-fufficiency, fo frequently become the dupes of their own imaginary fuperiority and indifcretion.

If the caufe had been inflammatory, arifing from the vifible effect of *plenitude, vifcidity*, or *grofs impurities* in the habit, the various evacuations might have been rotationally adopted, and juftified upon the principles of *rational* practice and medical confiftency; but unfortunately, in the prefent inftance, whatever tended to reduce the fyftem and diffolve the craffamentum of the blood, inevitably encreafed the very evil they were endeavouring to mitigate. It was equally remarkable and extraordinary, that no one article was brought into ufe but what became additionally injurious to the caufe it was intended to ferve; all which might have been

been prevented by the precaution of minutely infpecting, and properly comprehending, the *crafis of the blood*; the indifpenfible neceffity of which, I am anxioufly induced to hope, will acquire fuch weight with thofe who are adequate to the tafk of decifion, that it will in future become a bufinefs of more gene- ral inveftigation.

The repeated *bleedings*, the reduction of *aliment*, the perpetual adminiftration of *nitre*, (attenuating the blood that was before too ferous and watery) the injudicious interpo- fition of *purges*, and laftly, the infertion of the *rowel* to affift in the general devaftation, certainly exceeds every idea that could have been formed of random quackery and bodily depredation; this is, however, no more than *one* reprefentation of what is eternally carry- ing on in different places under the infpec- tion of thofe, who are too illiterate to poffefs a confiftent opinion of *their own*, and too im- pertinently conceited to folicit affiftance from *others*.

Defpairing of fuccefs by any relief that could be obtained from medicine, I or- dered

dered the fyftem to be immediately invigo-
rated with increafed fupplies of food, that by
forming the means of nutrition, the craffamentum of the blood might be augmented ;
affifting this with a pectoral cordial ball every
morning, not more to enliven the circulation,
than by warm and gentle ftimulation to re-
ftore the tone of the ftomach and inteftines,
totally debilitated by the injudicious adminiftration of *mercurial cathartics*, aud the long
and improper ufe of the *nitre*. Thefe defirable points being obtained, I recommended,
at the end of fix or feven days, the fair trial
of a courfe of the advertifed ALTERATIVE
POWDERS, to gradually obtund the acrimonious particles of the blood, with the
external application of the *Vegeto Mineral*,
properly proportioned to allay the irritation ; but I muft confefs, without any great
hope of fucceeding in parts of the frame
fo very remote from the active power of
medicine.

The other was the cafe of a COACH
HORSE, little lefs fingular in its mode of
treatment ; as no one ftep taken feemed to
be

be at all regulated by any well-founded in-tention of utility. The eyes (one more par-ticularly) had been some months in a state of failure and fluctuation, alternately pro-ducing hope and despair; when, after un-dergoing every experiment at home without even a probability of success, he was con-signed to my inspection, with a desire that I would be very minute in my instructions, which should be implicitly obeyed. Upon examination, I discovered the defect to have taken its seat in the humours of the eye, with no external inflammation attending, nor any other predominant trait than a dull cloudy aspect of the entire orb; displaying a pearly tint upon the outer edge of the cornea, surrounded by the tunica sclerotis, indicating the great probability of *film* and *opacity*, constituting in its gradual termination *total blindness*.

This horse I found, upon enquiry, had been treated in a way nearly similar to what we have just described; for having been repeatedly *bled and purged*, he had been subsisted upon *hot mashes*, and fur-nished with *four ounces of nitre* a day in his

his water for weeks together; had received the farrier's operative contribution of a *rowel*; and, to fum up the total of empirical fpeculation, and to verify the vulgar adage of " *the more cooks, &c.*" the meffenger (who was the commanding officer in the ftabularian department) CONFIDENTIALLY entrufted me with a *fecret* remedy of his own he had *privately* adopted; " the propriety and fafety of which application, he did not at all doubt but I fhould applaud, as it was, in general, *a perfect cure for bad eyes of every kind*; and was no more than TWO OUNCES OF BLUE VITRIOL diffolved in a quart of *fpring water*, with which the eyes were to be well wafhed every night and morning." Whatever may be my inclination, however highly I may be again difpofed to animadvert upon thefe acts of *defperation* or *madnefs*, (for fo I muft be permitted to term them) I fhall here drop the curtain upon the invincible ignorance and cruelty of this practice; referring the reader to various parts of the former volume, where he will be amply furnifhed with obfervations at large, perfectly applicable to the mode of treatment

9

ment fo ridiculoufly adapted to the cafes in queftion.

Not entertaining the leaft doubt but upon thefe reprefentations, by much the greater part of the judicious and enlightened world will perfectly coincide with me in an opinion not be eradicated ; that numbers of horfes annually lofe not only their *eyes* but their *lives*, by the dreadful effects of unbounded ignorance and confidence ; that it is to be lamented, too frequently act in conjunction, to the palpable prejudice of undifcerning credulity. Confidering this a fact too fubftantial to be fhaken by fpeculative or inexperienced opinions, it becomes for the completion of our purpofe, abfolutely neceffary we advert to the mifchiefs fo frequently occafioned by the fafhionable and indifcriminate ufe of *nitre*, in confequence of the general encomiums of former writers, before its properties were fo critically afcertained ; which added to the pecuniary eafe of acquifition, has brought the article into too great a degree of conftant ufe, in almoft every cafe, without a relative confideration to its medical property, the caufe

or

8

or symptoms of disease, its injurious tendency in some cases, or evident destruction in others, as in the former of the two just described.

That the frequent *use* and *abuse* of NITRE may not only be better understood but more perfectly retained in memory; as well as to establish the propriety of its use in *some cases*, and to confirm the justice of my assertion respecting its prejudicial effects *in others*; I must be under the necessity of introducing the repetition of a few lines descriptive of its properties, so particularly enlarged upon in my former volume, where it may be found by reference to the index. In animadversion upon the *unlimited* eulogiums of BARTLET, who has, without proper discrimination, recommended its frequent use to " *three or four ounces three times a day*," I have said,

" He urges the administration of it to attenuate and thin the dense sizy blood during the effect of inflammatory fever; this property of attenuation being allowed, what must be the natural conclusion and consequence of giving it in such large proportions? **Why** every *professional man*, knowing the mode by which it must inevitably affect the circulation, would naturally expect it to dissolve the very craffamentum of the blood, and reduce it to an absolute *serum* or aqueous vapour."

Admitting this reprefentation of its analized properties to stand incontroverted, what must prove its evident effects upon the *crafis of the blood*, already too much impoverished for " the standard of mediocrity neceffary to the prefervation of health?" and how diftreffingly erroneous must have been its introduction and continuance, in the former cafe of the two we have recited! to elucidate its destructive tendency in which, the prefent repetition of its defcription is particularly applied.

It is abfolutely aftonishing how very much *time*, affifted by the torrent of popular impreffion, may pervert the best intentions to the worst of purpofes; this has been fo truly the cafe in the frequent proftitution of this medicine. that little need be introduced to

insure

infure its credibility. NITRE is the general arcanum for every ill, while one-half of thofe who prefcribe, and the other half who give it, may be equally ftrangers to its effects or mode of operation. If a horfe is attacked with cold from an obftruction of the pores, that has thrown the perfpirable matter upon the eyes, lungs, or glandular parts, what is the eftablifhed remedy? *Nitre!* Inflammatory fever enfues, what follows? *Nitre!* Swelled legs, cracked heels, or greafe? *Nitre!* Bad eyes (from whatever caufe)? *Nitre!* In fact, fuch is the predominant rage of fafhionable phrenzy, that fhould any cafe arife, bearing in experience no pathognomonic fymptoms to afcertain the certainty or probable affinity of difeafe, its origin or termination, NITRE, with *fagacious grooms* and *condefcending farriers,* muft become the grand fpecific; to which infatuation, I am much inclined to believe BARTLET's unbounded partiality, and its *echo* from one *conjurer to another,* has very much contributed.

A chain of attentive obfervations, collected in the courfe of long experience, has fully

R 2

justified

juſtified me in a former opinion, that numerous injuries are ſuſtained, and ills inflicted, upon horſes of gentlemen by the ha-
zardous experiments of grooms and ſervants ;
who piqueing themſelves upon heterogeneous and ſelf-planned compoſitions or obſolete
preſcriptions, encreaſe danger or promote
deſtruction without detection. And what
renders the buſineſs a matter of more ſerious conſideration, is the unaccountable ob-
ſtinacy, pride, and *ſtabularian conſequence*
(of all other the moſt diſguſting) annexed to
their *affected knowledge* and *phyſical penetra-*
tion. Too ignorant to be convinced, and too
rude to become ſubſervient, expoſtulation or
explanation can hold no weight in the ſcale
of converſation ; conſequently no reformation can be expected in ſuch infernal ſyſtem
of domeſtic deception and deſtructive quackery, unleſs gentlemen, for the promotion of
their own intereſt and the ſafety of their
ſtuds, will condeſcend to exert their authority, and aboliſh a cuſtom in the encouragement or permiſſion of which they are ſo
materially injured. To the eſtabliſhment of
this fact, a numerous catalogue of moſt
ſubſtantial proofs are within my own know-

ledge,

ledge, was their communication of the leaft utility, in confirming an affertion that will, I believe, be readily admitted by all the world without exception.

From fuch medical remarks as unavoidably branch directly from the fubject, we return to exercife; the great importance of which cannot be too perfectly underftood, or regularly perfevered in for the prefervation of health. Having, I believe, properly defined the phyfical effects of gradual motion, fo far as it appertains to the animal œconomy in fecretion and excretion, (with its confequent advantages in air and exercife) it becomes neceffary to introduce fuch general rules as eftablifh the bafis of regular exercife, although the *time* and *manner* muft ever be regulated by the temper and caprice of the parties, feafon of the year, fituation, weather, and other contingencies not to be governed by the privilege of the pen, or the power of the prefs.

The apology for, or rather burlefque upon, the exercife of horfes (or more properly invalids) in the livery ftables of London,

R 3   is

is evidently calculated to complete the measure of mifery fo fully explained in our
laſt chapter, particularly in the winter feafon; that it is neceſſarily a matter of previous confideration to fuch inſtructions as
we may hereafter introduce under this head.
The poor animals I now allude to, ſeem
to exiſt as an almoſt different ſpecies to
thoſe enjoying the inexpreſſible advantages
of *country air, ſtrong exerciſe, and rural*
management. Here you perceive all ſpirit,
animation, and vigour, with both the horſes
and their attendants : in the metropolis, bodily infirmities and debilitation with one;
idleneſs, deception, ſloth, and *dejection* with
the other. In fact, the cauſes and effects
have been fo perfectly clear in the gantlet
of perſonal infpection and pecuniary experience, when the prevalence of faſhion
(or rather folly) influenced me to keep
two in ſuch ſituation, that no inducement
whatever ſhould prevail on me to leave
a horſe of the leaſt value open to the inconveniencies of ſuch ſtate for twenty-four
hours; perfectly convinced he would have
every probable chance of fuſtaining greater
injuries than might be obliterated in twice
twenty-

twenty-four days.   The more we inveftigate this bufinefs, the lefs fatisfaction it will afford to the parties more immediately in-terefted in the explanation ; particularly to thofe whofe fituations in life, or profef-fional avocations, leave them without an al-ternative.

After taking a retrofpective view of the " STABLING" already defcribed, let it be remembered, that what they call *exercife* depends entirely upon the inclination and convenience of the *motley crew* to whom the management of the. yard, and fuper-intendance of the horfes are entrufted ; thefe are a fort in general felected as the greateft adepts in falfhood and impofition, beft adapted to the convenient purpofes of the mafter, and the purified principles of a ftable-yard proficiency.   When fuch ex-ercife is, however, correfponding with the *inclination* and *convenience* of the parties we defcribe ; obferve in *its manner* how little it is calculated to promote the very purpofes for which it is intended.

The horfe is brought in general from the

R 4

evapo-

evaporating 'fteams of the moft volatile falts, with the perfpirative pores all open, parch-ing with thirft, to a large open trough of cold water, (with little refpect to feafon) where he is permitted to fatiate the appetite, unreftrained by judgment or fear of confe-quence ; till chilled by the frigidity of the element, the porous fyftem becomes in-ftantly collapfed, and you perceive by at-tention, the tail almoft immediately clung to the hind quarters ; a violent trembling and bodily agitation fucceeds, and the perfpira-tive matter thus obftructed in its *very act of fluctuation*, (through every part of the frame) lays the foundation of various ills, that however they might have been avoided in the firft inftance, cannot be prevented in the laft.

This ceremony is fucceeded by one of two others equally prejudicial to the frame in general, however its ill effects may not prove immediately difcernable ; but remain dormant fome fhort fpace of time in the habit before it is difplayed in one of the many difeafes fo repeatedly defcribed in different parts of the laft and prefent chap-ters.

ters. For fo foon as the horfe has been thus permitted to glut himfelf with an immoderate quantity of the cold water beforementioned, he is directly configned *to his ftall*, where its injurious effects are prefently vifible in a fevere rigor, or violent fit of fhaking, not unlike the painful paroxyfm of an intermittent ; producing an almoft inftantaneous contraction of the cutaneous paffages, and "ftaring of the coat," (as it is called) when we obferve,

> " Each particular Hair to ftand on End
> " Like Quills upon the fretful Porcupine."

The alternative to this practice is fo thoroughly contemptible, that it is abfolutely difficult to decide which is the moft deftructive or dangerous of the two; for if the plan above-defcribed is not adopted, but at times admits of variation, it is directly in the following way : The horfe thus watered, is immediately mounted by one of the *juvenile ragamuffins*, who conftantly give daily attendance at thofe receptacles, to obtain a proficiency in the arts of *riding, cruelty,* and *perfecution*. Two or three of the horfes at a time, and in

this

this ftate, are put into a courfe of exercife, and *woeful exercife* it certainly is with
a witnefs; for without the leaft previous
gentle walking, to expedite the gradual
evacuation of excrements fo long retained
for want of motion, they are inftantly trotted, gallopped, and perpetually turned at
each end of a fhort ride, in fuch fcene of inceffant confufion for a length of time without remiffion. The ftomach and inteftines
being over-loaded with their contents, the
horfe is totally inadequate to rapidity of
motion without great bodily diftrefs; a few
minutes therefore puts him into a wonderful
degree of perfpiration; when evidently labouring under a difficulty of refpiration and
difquietude, he is returned tottering to the
ftable, and there left to grow " cool at lei-
fure;" laying, *in another way*, the foundation of thofe difeafes refulting from a collapfion of the porous fyftem, and ftagnation of
perfpirable matter, too fubftantial to be reforbed into the circulation.

Taking leave for the prefent of ftable
difcipline, fo truly defpicable that farther
descrip-

defcription might be confidered a proftitution of both time and paper, we neceffarily return to the gradations of exercife
beft adapted to the different degrees of
horfes, according to their various ftates of
condition. Many calculations have been
made upon the poffible labour and continued exertions of this fpecies, and we are
by no means ignorant of their great and
almoft incredible execution, when brought
(for the decifion of bets) into trials of feverity upon the *turf* or *road*, both in fpeed and
duration.

The diftinction to be made in the prefent inftance, is only the line between what
is to be confidered as *work*, and what as
the falutary intervention of *exercife*; opinions (fo near as fpeculative attention can
form a degree of confiftency) admit, that
horfes of moderate qualifications and moderately fupported, will conftantly travel, or
journey in their accuftomed employment,
from fixteen to twenty miles *every day*,
through the year, without the leaft inconvenience or bodily debilitation, more than
what naturally arifes from the increafing age
of

of the fubject. This, however, being fixed
as a kind of conditional ftandard, or general
criterion, cannot be fuppofed to be held *critically correct* with all horfes, without diftinction; as there are many that will confequently
bear much more labour and fatigue, from
greater bodily ftrength, inherent fpirit, or
conftitutional ftamina, than others that fall
very far fhort in conftant work and execution,
from a want of thofe perfections fo truly valuable in horfes of the former defcription.

As I have before faid, exercife, in all its
particulars of *manner, diftance,* and *duration,*
muft be entirely regulated by contingent reflections upon the *health, ftate,* and *condition*
of the fubject; fo it muft be perfectly clear,
that the recommendation of certain exercife
to horfes in a high ftate of health and condition, cannot be fuppofed to extend to thofe
under phyfic, or in different ftates of, or recovery from, difeafe: Such muft unavoidably receive judicious regulations from the
parties concerned; as the kind of daily exercife we now have in contemplation, only
appertains to horfes in health, the prefervation of which is the prefent object of confideration.

fideration. All the obfervations under this head, having been introduced to demonftrate the UTILITY OF EXERCISE IN GENERAL, and the *ills* that certainly arife from *the want of it*, more than to lay down fpecific rules for the daily exercife of particular horfes; fuch inftructions will be found included under the management of HUNTERS and ROAD HORSES, when we come to enlarge upon thofe different heads.

R O W E L L I N G

H A S been to the credulous and illiterate of *paft times*, exactly what the fafcinating infatuation of ANIMAL MAGNETISM proves to the dupes of the *prefent*; like HUMOURS, it has been played upon by moft writers in rotation, without an explanatory line in its favour to produce fatisfactory *proof* of its mechanical procefs or eftablifhed utility. BRACKEN, who hardly ever gave caufe of complaint for abridging his fubject, but generally moft condefcendingly fpun it (by a variety of branches) to *an almoft indivifible thread*, deviated in this inftance from his ufual cuftom; and after introducing

troducing the fubject with a certain degree of dignity annexed to its importance, by telling us, " he once thought not to have made a particular chapter upon rowelling," he *begins* and *concludes* that very chapter, of fo much confequence, in the *fingle duodecimo page* 321, of his firft volume. In this page, and upon this bufinefs, I had very much wifhed to have enlarged my own ideas, and improved my judgment; more particularly, upon the abftrufe effects of a fubject, whofe perfonal or literary advocates have been *hitherto* enabled to advance but little in profeffional fupport of their favourite operation.

To obtain fatisfactory information and fyftematic knowledge upon the efficacy of ROWELS, when judicioufly inferted, I have been for years ftudioufly induftrious to better my opinion by the moft inquifitive attention to every *attempt at definition*, from thofe who were remarkable for their extenfive practice to thofe who were no lefs fingular for their illiteracy; in anxious hope that *time*, or *circumftance*, might contribute more to a gratification of my wifh than my expectation. To avoid troubling the Reader

Reader with tedious or unneceffary quotations, I fhall let it fuffice to introduce fuch
abbreviations only as become perfectly applicable to our future remarks upon the fubject before us.

BRACKEN juftly obferves, " Rowelling is
the common refource of Farriers in general;
amongft whom, he could never find one that
could give a fatisfactory account of the *ufe* or
abufe; but they all tell you, a rowel is to
draw off the bad or corrupt humours from
the blood; and this is to cure almoft every
diforder, according to their way of reafoning." This affertion is fo ftrictly true, that
I will cheerfully confent to its confirmation,
upon the experimental enquiries of the laft
twenty years; and declare, I never could
acquire from the *Vulcanian profeffors*, a more
technical or enlightened defcription of the
OPERATIVE EFFECTS, than the " *poor epitome*" he acknowledges to have received.

In this communication there is nothing
very extraordinary; but it is not fo in what
is to follow, and is worthy obfervation. In the
fame page, and almoft the next line, he tells

us, " it is good in a great many difeafes ;"
and inftantly fays : " The horfe might as
well, náy better, lofe as much *blood* every
day as he does *matter* by the *rowel*; for it is
as certainly blood as that in the veins, barring
the colour, which makes no effential difference ; and he is very much of opinion that
feveral cures are wholly attributed to *rowelling*, when reft and patience are the principal inftruments or agents that perform it."

Is there any one reader who will not be
greatly furprifed, and as highly entertained,
when he is informed that the writer, who
has recommended the ufe of rowels for the
cure of various difeafes, in compliance with
the force of that very cuftom he condemns,
fhould in the fame page, and comparatively
with the fame breath, inftantly reprobate the
practice, as abfolutely drawing fo much *blood*
from the *veins* ; poffeffing at the fame time
fo great a verfatility of literary genius, fo perfect a pantomimic tranfpofition of words and
opinions, that we find him (p. 85.) prefcrib-
ing " bleeding, purging, and rowelling *in
feveral places at once*, for one rowel is of
little avail for many reafons ; and thefe fhould
continue

continue running a confiderable time, at leaft a fortnight or three weeks." In page 99, he believes they may be ufeful in many difor-ders, " provided there be made *a fufficient number of them* ;" but as to the parts of the body, whether behind the ears, in the breaft, or under the horfe's belly, he thinks it is much the fame thing ; " for in reality, they are no more than adding a number of *anus's* or *fundaments*, fo that NATURE may meet with them in feveral parts of the body, and not be put to the trouble of going the more tedious and common round of circulation in order for a difcharge by *excrement* or *dung*."

Can it be poffibly neceffary for me to offer a fingle line in apology for the introduction of affertions fo exceedingly oppofite from the fame pen ; or a *refinement of thought* and *fublimity of language* in the latter, not to be exceeded by any hypothetical reafoning or fer-tility of invention ever iffued from the prefs ? The idea of *artificial fundaments*, to fave NA-TURE the trouble of going the more tedious and common road by the *anus*, is not only fo truly great and inimitable ; fo very contrary to and fo far furpaffing the affertion of OSMER,

VOL. II. S that

that " the works of the Divine Artift" had left no room for rectification ; (fee p. 153) that nothing on my part can be required to excite the rifible emotions ; though, I muft confefs, it is with the greateft reluctance fo fair a temptation is relinquifhed, to play a little upon the retentive imperfections of one predeceffor, and the methodiftical enthufiafm of the other.

But notwithftanding the direct and repeated contradictions we find difperfed through the volumes of BRACKEN, (probably occafioned by his long and inconfiftent digreffions) it muft be acknowledged, with the ftricteft adherence to juftice and merit, that no one fucceeding writer has fince ftarted a thought or broached an opinion upon the operation of rowelling, or its effects, but what has been an exact literal defcription, or *oblique echo,* of what originated with him upon the fubject. For upon a minute examination of the various publications of different writers, we find that a very fuperficial inveftigation, and no additional explanation, has been condefcendingly beftowed upon a procefs that is even now held in the higheft eftimation, by

2

thofe

thofe advocates for ancient practice, who can communicate no fcientific or profeffional defcription of its operative effect upon the conftitution; or by what phyfical means the improvement is to be obtained, that they fo confidently and *confcientioufly* recommend upon every poffible occafion.

The very few lines introduced under this head, by even the moft prolific authors, poffefs not the leaft ray of novelty or inftruction, but are direct imitations of what proceeded from BRACKEN; beginning with the cuftomary remark, " that rowels are in general ufe, but little underftood;" " that they are artificial vents between the fkin and the flefh;" " that they act by revulfion and derivation;" carrying off the redundant HUMOURS from the veffels by *depletion*.

Thefe few paffages contain in purport the whole that has been at all communicated through the medium of the prefs, upon an operation fo indifcriminately recommended in almoft every difeafe without exception; notwithftanding it is of fo much

S 2

confequence

confequence in medical management, that it becomes matter of admiration, how the enlightened part of the world can be fo frequently made the dupes of a moft confummate ignorance; without fummoning to their affiftance an opinion of their own, to juftify the confiftency or prevent the error of fuch proceeding. For my own part, after endeavouring moft induftrioufly for many years, to fathom the depth of a *Farrier's* intellectual and profeffional abilities, without being enabled to place any part to their *credit accompt*; and conftantly drawing a mental comparifon between the *good* they might *poffibly do*, and the mifchief they would *certainly occafion*, I have long fince found it neceffary to decline every dependence upon either: feeling myfelf perfectly juftified in recommending it moft heartily to every reader poffeffing the leaft attachment to the fpecies; never to fuffer a medicine to be given, or an operation to be performed, before the expected procefs of the former, and the intentional effect of the latter are previoufly explained to his entire fatisfaction.

This

This I am the more readily induced to do, by the inceſſant inſertion of rowels and adminiſtration of drinks, by parties ſo confeſſedly ignorant, they can never aſſign the leaſt reaſon for the operative ſucceſs of one, or the expected medical relief from the other. It is not long ſince I became an accidental ſpectator to a caſe of great danger and almoſt immediate diſſolution, when the horſe was in the ſlings nearly exhauſted, with only a few hours to live ; and was conſequently very much ſurpriſed to hear a Farrier of faſhionable local eminence, earneſtly recommend and attempt to proceed to the inſertion of a multiplicity of rowels, (that were however not permitted by the owner) ; when the horſe was inevitably doomed to death long before the rowels could have taken any other effect, than in their conſequent inflammation (previous to maturation) to have encreaſed his miſery and rendered his laſt moments the more excruciating. However, if the owner had conſented, the operations would have been performed, and the reward expected, conſequently *ſome purpoſe* anſwered.

I con-

I confidered myfelf exceedingly lucky, in fo favourable an opportunity, to acquire fome-thing perfonally fatisfactory upon the ope-rative procefs and probable effect of rowels upon the frame and habit, from one who had fo confidently recommended their im-mediate ufe in a cafe of fo much emer-gency ; and really expected, from the ex-tenfive practice of the party and the gene-ral acknowledgement of his practical abili-ties, that I fhould have been in a propor-tional degree gratified ; but forry I am to confefs, after every direct attack, oblique infinuation, and crofs examination, he was fo well *fortified in his entrenchments,* that I could derive no greater degree of informa-tion than " they were the *likelieft things* to do him good."

This, among many other recommenda-tions of rowelling, upon foundations equally ridiculous, brings to my mind another in-ftance of the indifcriminate ufe of rowels, with no other reafon on earth than a felf-interefted reference to the pecuniary com-penfation annexed to the ceremony of opera-tion.   A few weeks fince, an intimate friend calling upon me one morning, informed me, he he had met with an unlucky circumftance; for having unexpectedly fold his horfe on the Saturday at READING, without any previous intention of fo doing, he was by agreement to be delivered on the Monday morning; at which time the purchafer difcovering a violent inflammation and difcharge from one of the eyes, (which was not in that condition at the time of purchafe) he objected to receiving him; but its being concluded the temporary effect of a *bite, blow,* or *cold,* he at length agreed to take him away, with the privilege of returning him at any time *within a week,* if fuch appearance was not entirely removed. This not happening, the horfe was returned; and my friend had then left him in the hands of the *fmith,* (or FARRIER) who had that moment taken away two quarts of blood, and was, when he came away, juft going to put in *a rowel* below the breaft, to draw off the HUMOUR that was fettled in the eye; that he had alfo recommended the ufe of *nitre* and *fulphur:* and as he had *plenty at home,* he fhould give him an ounce of each, night and morning.

S 4 The

The rapid accumulation and combination of remedies naturally excited fome expoftulation, and influenced me to afk, whether there were any predominant reafons (exclufive of the interefted recommendation of the operator) that induced him fo foon to permit the infertion of the rowel, before he had waited even *twenty-four hours*, to obferve whether any advantage had been derived from the bleeding, which was certainly the firft and beft ftep that could have been taken ? Finding alfo, upon minute enquiry, that there was a great probability of its having been occafioned by a bite or blow among other horfes, when replaced in the ftable, between the time of his having been agreed for and brought away ; I prevailed on him to poftpone the rowel, (which he had but juft time to do, as the incifion was made before his return) relinquifh his *nitrous, fulphureous* intention for the prefent, and leave his horfe in my ftable ; which having cheerfully complied with, the eye was perfectly found and clear in a few days, with no other affiftance than a flight wafhing twice a day with a fponge, plentifully impregnated with cold fpring water.

This

This circumftance, of very little confequence in itfelf, is introduced to corroborate the affertion, that rowels are frequently
and injudicioufly brought into practice, without reafon in the operator, or reflection in
the owner; who generally alarmed upon
every flight occafion, feizes the firft twig of
confolation, without giving the matter fuch
confideration as would enable him to recollect every *probable remedy* fhould have REA-
SON for its foundation; upon the *profpect* of
which he would certainly be, in moft cafes,
as capable of deciding as his SCIENTIFIC
INSTRUCTOR. But what renders the recital of fo trivial a bufinefs applicable to our
prefent purpofe is, the expeditious cure that
muft inevitably have been attributed to the
ROWEL, with no fmall portion of collateral merit to thofe ufeful auxiliaries, the
fulphur and *nitre*, had they been (luckily for
the advifer) concerned in a work, that NA-
TURE would fo frequently perform by her
own efforts, if not inceffantly counteracted
by thofe who neither comprehend her œconomy, nor condefcend to confult her indications.

I   Having

Having introduced what became abfolutely unavoidable, to demonftrate the frequent abfurdity (from long ftanding, and invincible cuftom) of applying rowels in many cafes, without the leaft well founded reafon for their ufe ; it becomes neceffary to difcover, by fcientific enquiry, what can be advanced in proof of the fuppofed utility, that has for ages rendered them the profeffional (*or political*) rage of every clafs of EQUESTRIAN DOCTORS, without diftinction. BRACKEN, as I have before obferved, fays, he attributed much of the virtue of rowelling to the good effects of *reft* and *patience*; and I am not a little vain that we fall into a direct coincidence of opinion upon fo principal a part of the fubject.

Previous to the intended inveftigation of their operative procefs and effects, I cannot but exprefs my difappointment in not finding fomething more fatisfactory from the very intelligent and much enlightened pen of Mr. Clarke, to whofe profeffional merits I fhall ever be one of the firft to fubfcribe ; though unluckily upon this head, he has not defcanted with his wonted perfpicuity, but very

much

much contracted his usual portion of information; not condescending to bestow a chapter of more than *five short pages*, merely to explain the mechanical part of the operation, the places proper for insertion, an insinuation of the probable danger, and lastly, as every writer has done before, boldly asserted their universal excellence, without a single substantial proof, upon which their reputed efficacy can be judiciously founded.

" Rowels (says he) are of great use in carrying off rheums or defluxions from the eyes; in great swellings of the glands, &c. about the throat and jaws, which threaten a suffocation; or when the head seems particularly affected, as in the vertigo, or staggers, apoplexy, &c. &c. in recent lameness; swellings of the legs and heels, attended with a discharge of thin ichorous matter, &c. in large and sudden swellings in any part of the body; or when extravasations of the fluids have taken place from blows, bruises, &c. or when a horse has had a severe fall, &c. and

in

in a variety of other cafes, which will occur to the judicious practitioner."

Without indulging the leaft defire or intention to animadvert with feverity upon the different writers who have thus rotationally reprefented the accumulated perfection of rowels, (that feem in their progrefs for the laft century, to have acquired, like the *noftrums* of the prefent day, the virtues of curing all difeafes) it is very natural to conclude, that the above lift, in each of which they are faid to be "of great ufe," with the repeated introduction of "et ceteras," and the variety of "other cafes fubmitted to the judicious practitioner," that there can be but *very few,* or in fact, *none,* to which they are not, in the opinions of *fome,* perfectly applicable *in one way or another,* perhaps in no one more than the felf-evident confolation, if it does *no good* it may do *no harm!* it will at any rate fupport the appearance of bufinefs! If NATURE effects her own purpofe and promotes a *cure,* the rowel will be entitled to a portion of credit, and the operator

rator to no fmall fhare of profeffional reputation.

Thefe are privileges againft the power of which there can be no appeal; but if we look into the operative procefs of rowels with the eye of accuracy, and advert to their origin, we fhall find they were introduced at a period much lefs enlightened; when the great efficacy of ALTERATIVES was but little, if at all known or eftablifhed to any degree of certainty, more particularly to thofe who are generally entrufted with the medical fuperintendance of horfes; that however expert or judicious they may prove in the operative parts of FARRIERY, muft feel themfelves exceedingly mortified at knowing nothing of medicines, their origin, preparations, combinations, properties, or effects.

This univerfal deficiency fo generally admitted, to which the major part of their profeffional errors may be juftly attributed, now bids fair to be refcued from its difgraceful ftate of barbarifm, (under which ftigma it has fo long laboured) by a plan
that

that is foon to be fubmitted to Parliament by the ODIHAM AGRICULTURE
SOCIETY, who have already made public
(and folicited fubfcriptions for the promotion of) their very laudable intention of
fending a certain number of youths annually to FRANCE for VETERINARIAN EDU-
CATION : Though it perhaps reflects no
great degree of credit upon our own nation, that a ftill more laudable plan could
not have been adopted, by laying the
foundation ftone of fuch inftitution in this
kingdom ; where, by the means of inftruction being local and more extenfive, the
advantages muft certainly become the fooner
general, than under the reftraints of the
prefent propofition. For the very limited
number (I believe *four* or *fix*) that they
intend fending annually, under the uncertainty of pecuniary contribution from the
purfes of individuals, affords every reafon
to fuppofe, upon the moft moderate computation, that it muft be at leaft A CEN-
TURY before the good effect of fo defirable an improvement can be *univerfally*
experienced. But as every ftep to general
reformation muft have obftacles of much
magni-

magnitude to furmount, under the confola-
tory adage of " better *late* than *never*," every
member of the community muft wifh it the
moft uninterrupted fuccefs.

Returning to the operative part of our
fubject, and its falutary effects upon the
conftitution, it may be remembered, that
rowels have been ftrenuoufly recommended by advocates of every denomination, to
draw off the corrupt or difeafed HUMOURS
from *the blood*, leaving the remainder in a
ftate of purification ; this, however, has
never been roundly and boldly afferted as
a fact not to be difputed, but founded originally in conjecture, and pufillanimoufly
reiterated accordingly. But for the moment, and better promotion of difquifition
and the difcovery of truth, let us admit
the abfurdity ; out of which will evidently
arife a queftion to eftablifh the fallacy of
opinion founded in *error*, and foftered by
ignorance ; *viz.* Whether any profeffional
writer, or fcientific inveftigator, will ftand
forth and fay, the operative effect of a
rowel is equally applicable to the difference of difeafe, arifing from either a VIS-
CID

CID TENACITY; or an *acrimonious* and *impoverished* ſtate of the blood?

For the preceding quotation from CLARKE, (which is in fact a quotation from all the reſt) evidently recommends it in a variety of diſorders reſulting from *each* of the *two*; and ſhould ſuch ſyſtem poſſeſs the happy influence of extracting (ſecundem artem) the foundation of diſeaſes clearly proceeding from properties in the blood *ſo directly oppoſite to each other,* and ſuch wonderful efficacy can be ſubſtantially corroborated; I ſhall cheerfully become a convert to the prevalent opinion of the Vulcanian fraternity, and join in their unlimited repreſentation of GENERAL UTILITY. But till better and more profeſſional allegations are produced, to juſtify the indiſcriminate hold they have ſo long retained, (particularly in country practice); I ſhall conſcientiouſly forbear to contribute a ſingle encomium upon the great and almoſt infallible virtues they have been ſo univerſally and erroneouſly *ſuppoſed* to poſſeſs.

All

All opinions have not only agreed, but experience has eſtabliſhed the fact, that the matter diſcharged from the rowels, is, as BRACKEN has firſt obſerved, " as certainly *blood* as that in the veins, barring the colour." This is re-aſſerted by every ſucceeding author, and can admit of no contrariety of opinion tending to cavil or controverſy ; being a matter profeſſionally fixed beyond the poſſibility of either. What inference then is conſequently to be drawn from this admiſſion ? Why, that every part of the circulation, both in quantity and quality, contributes equally to that very diſcharge ſo ridiculouſly ſuppoſed to conſiſt of the *diſeaſed portion* only ; when the inſertion has been as erroneouſly fixed upon or near to ſome particular part, to be intentionally relieved by the partial power of ſuch artificial evacuation ; conſtituting a ſecond blunder upon the palpable foundation of the former. For it muſt prove a diſgraceful proſtitution of even *common comprehenſion,* to indulge the leaſt idea, that a larger portion of craſſamentum or ſerum can individually undergo a greater change or rectification

VOL. II.   T   fication

fication in feparation and extravafation than the other.

It being therefore proved nothing more or lefs (divefted of technical terms and ambiguous reafoning) than a gradual depletion of the blood veffels, (divefted of its fanguinary appearance, and becoming matter by the natural procefs of extravafation and rarefaction) let us decifively pronounce what fuch conftant evacuation can be productive of in its effects; I believe I may venture to pronounce every profeffor of phyfic or farriery will perfectly agree with me, in confirming it nothing more than a certain mode of reducing the habit by drawing off a greater portion of blood in every twenty-four hours, than is generated by the nutritive property of the given quantity of aliment, allowed for fubfiftance in the fame fpace of time; though it is, *in all cafes*, ridiculoufly conceived, that by reducing the bodily ftrength, you infallibly fubdue the predominance of difeafe alfo.

We now arrive at the very line of diftinction neceffary to be drawn in all cafes,

5

where

where a rowel is, or can be fuppofed to become at all adequate to the tafk it is affigned. For inftance, in cafes arifing from caufes threatening inflammation, or fuch grofs impurities as are evidently the effect of a crude and vifcid ftate of the blood, (it being firft properly afcertained) they have moft certainly much in their favour upon the well-founded maxim before quoted, " if they do *no good,* they *may* do no harm ;" it is certainly no bad plan *in fporting* to obtain as many points as poffible in your favour : but as I will by no means recommend to the practice of others, what I would cautioufly avoid in my own ; I muft confefs they fhould never be brought into immediate ufe in ftables under my fuperintendance, till the more rational and mild methods of *Evacuants* and *Diuretics* (according to the nature, duration and feverity of the cafe) had been tried without probability or indications of fuccefs. And this idea of procraftination is held forth only upon what I term a very fufficient foundation ; for what man living, in poffeffion of free agency, and the happy power of reflection, would, after proper delibera-

tion,

tion, confent to perforate the hide of his horfe, and ftand the doubtful chances of complicated difquietude, a lucky formation and fortunate flow of matter; an ill-conditioned wound, inveterate ulcer, or prominent cicatrix, conftituting an irreparable blemifh, when it can be fo readily avoided?

But admitting, in compliment to ancient practice, their utility to be obvious in the inflammatory or vifcid cafes before recited; let us make a fair and candid enquiry into the lift of Mr. CLARKE's, not long fince quoted, (which is, in fact, BRACKEN's, BARTLET's, and OSMER's alfo) and openly acknowledge where it will be proper to coalefce, and where diffent from fuch opinions; that their *great and indifcriminate merit* may with propriety come before that public tribunal, to whofe decifive arbitration every *literary difquifitionift* muft ultimately fubmit.

That the fubject (and of importance it certainly is) may meet the eye and attract the judgment of every unbiaffed inveftigator

gator with all poffible clearnefs; it fhall be perfectly divefted of every ambiguity and remote confideration, by re-ftating fingly the cafes in which the different authors have fo lavifhly recommended their ufe; admitting the propriety of their intro-duction where their good effects become *probable* upon profeffional reafoning, or condemning the adoption where I feel myfelf juftified in fupporting a contrary opinion.

We are firft told, " Rowels are of great ufe in carrying off rheums or defluxions of the eyes;" but as no profeffional proofs have been adduced, or cafes authenticated, by any author whatever, to confirm *this opinion*, it is very natural to wifh for information, whether this " USE" has been afcertained *in effect*, with or without the affiftance of *cathartics*, *diuretics*, or *alteratives*, one of which, in thefe cafes, is generally called in to their affiftance : but as the effect of fuch medicines are not *externally perceptible*, their proportional fervices are buried in oblivion, (as not being brought totally to proof) and the glory of the victory, if obtained, is attri-

T 3

buted

buted to ROWELLING, as a favourite species of practice, not to be violated by the *rude* and *uncultivated* dictates of modern improvement. I must confess, in the cases we now speak of, I should by no means *too hastily* recommend their insertion ; but proceeding with a proper degree of consistency, according to the apparent cause from a state of the blood, prefer a course of *diuretics* or *alteratives,* (as the case might require) and reserve the operation of rowelling as my last resource, when every other method had failed of the expected success.

" In great swellings of the glands, &c. about the throat and jaws, which threaten a suffocation."—This is a recommendation so directly contrary to every systematic and scientific proceeding, that I shall confine both my surprize and remarks merely to a professional explanation ; and the introduction of my *own opinion,* in opposition *to theirs.* If the swellings were so alarming as to " threaten suffocation," and afforded no hope of speedy maturation, by topical applications, (which must ever prove the most

eligible

eligible and confiſtent method of relief) ſure-
ly *immediate*, *repeated*, and *occaſional* difcharges of blood, muſt contribute, in many
ways, to a removal of the danger appre-
hended, in cauſing ſome degree of revulſion
by depletion; which will undoubtedly, by
relieving the circulation, reduce the deſcribed
ſtricture upon the parts, and render ſuch proceeding very far preferable to the certain
hazard and tedious expectation of at *leaſt
three days*, for the bare chance of very ſlowly
counteracting what " ſuffocation" might prevent; long before one, or *a multiplicity of
rowels*, could arrive at a proper degree of
ſuppuration. And this is the very predominant reaſon why I think they are by no
means to be relied on in acute caſes of danger
and emergency; ſo much as repeated bleedings, and ſuch evacuations as become MORE
SPEEDILY effectual upon the frame and conſtitution.

" When the head ſeems particularly affected, as in the vertigo or ſtaggers, apoplexy,
&c. &c."——In theſe caſes, after proper bleedings, (which muſt precede every other conſideration) a proper examination of the blood,

T 4 and

and a neceffary removal of inteftinal obftruc-
tions, if they fhould be found requifite;
I cannot have the leaft objection to the infertion of a rowel, *or rowels*, provided the
patient (in either cafe) can be prevailed
upon to live *three or four days*, to try the
effect of the experiment; and this I admit
upon a recommendation in my former volume, that " increafing appearances of danger muft juftify exertions of alacrity and
fortitude :" Although I muft confefs my apprehenfion that either of the above cafes,
(unlefs early counteracted by the judicious
interpofition of other adminiftrations) muft
gain ground *too rapidly* upon the fyftem, to
undergo a fudden change of improvement,
by means fo very tardy in the effects of their
operation.

" In recent lamenefs."—Why in *recent*
lamenefs, and before any of the milder methods are introduced, I am at a lofs to conceive; but upon prefumption that every
other probable remedy is fet at defiance, for
the more applicable introduction of REST,
I ftart not the moft trifling objection, convinced it is the only plea that can be of-

6

fered

fered for the *inapplicable introduction* of the
ROWEL.

" Swelling of the legs and heels, attended with a difcharge of thin ichorous
matter, &c."—I imagine, in fuch cafe, the
rowel is meant to be inferted after a non-
fubmiffion to the entire claffes of *alteratives*
and *diuretics* ; whofe efficacious powers muft
be too well eftablifhed, by thofe who have
experienced their excellent properties, to be
entirely rejected, without fuch trial as they
are juftly entitled to by their rank in experimental practice.

" In large and fudden fwellings in any
part of the body."—This is a recommendation fo vague, loofe, and indefinite, that it
will hardly admit of conftruction or determination.   As " large and fudden fwellings"
may arife from various caufes, requiring very
different modes of treatment, it is natural to
conclude, (indeed to prove by practical demonftration) that *fudden* appearances muft
frequently juftify much MORE SUDDEN means
of counteraction, than patiently waiting, *day
after day*, for the expected and precarious
difcharge

difcharge of a rowel, that, after all the fuf-
pence, may probably terminate unfavourably,
to the lofs of the fubject and mortification
of the owner.

" When extravafations of the fluids have
taken place from blows, bruifes, &c."——Here
I cannot hefitate a moment to acquiefce in
the propofition, provided the infertion can
conveniently take place immediately *upon* or
clofe to the part affected : If that cannot be
done, I object to the attempt ; as the " ex-
travafated fluids" muft be abforbed into the
circulation before they can attain the place of
difcharge.   If which can be accomplifhed,
they may then be carried off by different
evacuants, without recourfe to fuch means ;
but if I perfectly comprehend the allufion,
it is fuppofed to convey an idea of " ex-
travafated fluids" become ftagnant by length
of time, and not to be reforbed into the circulation by any probable means whatever.
In which cafe the rowel may be adopted with
PROPRIETY, provided it is inferted under
the advantages I have juft defcribed ; that is,
directly *upon*, or immediately contiguous to,
the feat of difeafe.

" When

" When a horfe has had a fevere fall, &c. and in a variety of other cafes which will occur to the judicious practitioner."—This propofition covers fuch a wonderful *fcope of poffibility,* and includes fuch a variety of latitude for the enquirer ; that it is by far too unlimited in its comprehenfion to admit a tedious enumeration of remarks applicable to even *half the cafes* that may be brought into the fcale of imaginary probability. This will forcibly affect the judgment of every reader, if he condefcends, for a few moments only, to recollect the ways a horfe may be affected by a " fevere fall," are fo very numerous, that the advice here given (in fo extenfive a degree) muft prove conditionally dependant upon, and be regulated entirely by, the opinion of thofe to whom the fuperintendance of fuch cafes become fubject, rendering every farther remark upon this paffage extraneous and unneceffary.

After the ftricteft attention to, and inveftigation of this fyftem, (anciently adopted and tranfmitted, like domeftic property, or profeffional implements of *bellows, anvil, hammer,* and *vice,* from fire to fon) I feel impartially

impartially influenced to declare myfelf a very flender advocate for their continuance in practice upon the bafis of GENERAL UTI-LITY. There may be fome few cafes, and thofe few very confined in number, where, from a non-fubmiffion to the dictates of a more rational application, experiments may be made by the credulous, of their *fo univerfal reputation :* But I am induced moft heartily to believe, fuch alternative muft be adopted much more upon the conftruction of HOPE, than the too flattering profpect of EXPECTATION,

For my own part, voluntarily embarked in a conditional truft of honour with the public, for the promotion of equeftrian im-provements by every rational and fcientific means, that can be advanced upon the face of well-founded opinion or practical experience ; it is impoffible for me to acquiefce in the recommendation of their infertion, in the variety of indifcriminate cafes before recited ; from which I have withheld my approba-tion upon the firmeft conviction, that no fyftematic fubftantiated reafons have ever been promulgated, demonftrating the ope-rative

rative procefs upon the animal œconomy, from which the *reported good effects* are SUPPOSED TO BE PRODUCED.

I believe I have before hinted their being originally adopted in times of greater obfcurity; when the minds and manners were not only much lefs enlightened, but the almoft incredible property and power of medicine not then difcovered and brought palpably home, as it now is, to the moft obftinate incredulity. In the remote age of this invention, the volume of medical improvement might be juftly confidered in its infancy, emerging from the early efforts of antiquity; from which it has continued in gradual refinement to its prefent period of profeffional fplendor, under the indefatigable aufpices of thofe whofe literary additions to the works of fcience will perpetuate their memories very far beyond any effufions that can poffibly fall from the grateful pen of humble admiration.

It muft therefore fuffice in additional confirmation of the improvement we applaud, to obferve, that even in private practice amongft amongſt the human ſpecies, thoſe analogous operations, ISSUES and SETONS, in the courſe of the laſt forty or fifty years, are *comparatively obliterated*; bearing no kind of proportion in common uſe, being but very ſeldom either adviſed or adopted, but where the parties, from an invincible perſonal or *pecuniary* averſion to medicine, cannot be prevailed upon to undergo ſuch courſe as may evidently repair the *conſtitution*, to a certain partial *conſumption* of the purſe.

After every obſervation I have been able to deduce from theory, every remark I could collect in practice, and every information to be derived from thoſe VULCANIAN VETERINARIANS I have had the *honor to conſult;* after the analyzation of its phyſical proceſs upon the frame; its being immediately and equally fed from the fountain of circulation and ſupport; a proper inveſtigation and expoſure of the ridiculous idea of *partially* drawing off *corrupt* or *diſeaſed* particles from the blood, that the animal may " live the purer with the other half;" and laſtly, the more contemptible propagation of their being found applicable *to all diſeaſes,* without a ſingle

single professional proof manfully and scientifically demonstrated, that they are absolutely necessary or infallible IN ONE; it can create no admiration that I feel myself justified in offering to the world an opinion, very little subservient to the superficial decisions of those who have preceded me upon this subject.

Under the combined weight of these considerations, and so far as they entitle me to offer judgment, I dare venture to pronounce and promulgate such belief, that there are only a very few cases in which they are either individually *necessary* or *useful*; having it *at all* in their *effects*, the POWER to produce any such change in, or improvement upon, the constitution, but what may be more consistently (and to a greater certainty) produced by judicious interposition of *evacuants, diuretics, alteratives,* or such other class of medicines, as upon accurate investigation of the cause and reference to symptoms, may be found corresponding with the case and its explanatory parts, in our former volume, more particularly adapted to medical disquisition and the cure of disease.

The

The cafes to which they may be in fome degree adapted, bearing profeffional traits in their favour, are, partial fwellings of fome duration, originally occafioned by extrava- fated fluids become too vifcid by ftagnation to be reforbed into the circulation ; cuta- neous difeafes not fpeedily fubmitting to the courfe of medicines adapted to their peculiar clafs ; inveterate lamenefs of long ftanding in the fhoulders or ligamentary parts, by the retention of inflammatory matter firft fixed there by the improper and too free ufe of fpirituous applications ; and afthmatic complaints upon a confirmation of their non-fubmiffion to conditional bleedings, a moderate ufe of nitre, and fuch courfe of pectoral detergents as will be found re- commended under that head. In each of which, I fhould not hefitate a moment to urge the propriety of inferting the rowel as near the caufe of complaint as poffible ; that the flux of matter (though collected from the circulation) might flow directly from, or as contiguous to the feat as circumftances will permit ; and that fuch local infertion may contribute affiftance to whatever utility they poffefs, in unloading to a certainty
the

the neighbouring veffels concerned in the cafes we have juft defcribed. The advantage naturally refulting from fuch precaution becoming too evidently obvious to require farther anatomical defcription or phyfical difquifition ; the minutiæ of which, (fo far as it appertains to the operation in queftion) having been largely and accurately explained in the definition of HUMOURS, under the laft article of EXERCISE, and the prefent upon ROWELLING, cannot ftand in the leaft need of additional elucidation to render the whole perfectly intelligible to every comprehenfion.

H U N T E R S.

The particular management of horfes paffing under this denomination will appear to many matter of fo little confequence, that it muft create furprife how any thing *new* can be introduced upon a fubject *they conceive* fo univerfally and perfectly underftood. However fuch opinion may be eftablifhed in the contracted minds

of thofe who exift only in error, and never
condefcend to fanction the moft promifing
ray of improvement ; the great number of
valuable horfes that have loft their lives,
either in or immediately after the chace, in
the two laft feafons only, with his Majefty's,
his Royal Highnefs the Prince of Wales's,
Lord Barrymore's, and Captain Parker's
hounds, are demonftrative proofs of *inabi-
lity* in the grooms, or *indifcretion* in the
riders ; as well as collateral corroboration
that the fyftem of perfection is not yet attained even in the firft hunting ftables of
fafhion and eminence.

Without prefuming to arraign, in the
prefent inftance, the judgment of *one,* or
the prudence of the *other,* I fhall proceed
to lay down fuch rules for the felection of
hunters, and the minute particulars of their
management, as have for a feries of more
than twenty years enabled me to enjoy the
pleafures of the chace with a multiplicity
of the fleeteft and moft popular packs in
different parts of the kingdom ; without one
of thofe unlucky contingencies, that fo frequently throw lefs thinking, or lefs experienced

enced fportfmen into the back ground of the picture with mortification and dif-grace.

It fhould be indelible in the mind of every juvenile and recent fportfman, that to bring a horfe into the field *out of condition,* incurs inftantaneous *fufpicion,* if not con-tempt; the curiofity (not to fay infulting in-difference) of every fpectator is excited, who fortunately excels in the figure or qualifica-tions of his fteed, and the fuperiority of his equipments. And this is not at all to be wondered at, when thofe entirely unac-quainted with the fact are informed; that as much emulation is perceptible in the dif-play of a *fporting apparatus,* as in the exult-ing fplendor of a birth-day appearance in the vicinity of St. James's: not only the RIDERS, but their HORSES are fraught with the infectious fpirit of rivalfhip; and impatiently wait the moment, that infpires each with the vigour of general conten-tion.

Horfes imperfect in their appearance, with fulnefs of the legs, foulnefs in the coat, cracks

in

in the heels, or poverty in the frame, are immediately furveyed with the eye of attentive infpection; this *oblique* but *accurate* furvey as certainly terminates to the difcredit of the mafter as the prejudice of the fervant, leaving no favourable impreffion of their ftable management at home, or equeftrian prudence in the field.

External deficiency is not the only inconvenience arifing from improper condition; the concomitant ills refulting from it, are not unfrequently attended with the moft ferious confequences. Horfes for the very fevere and ftrong chaces with STAG or FOX, fhould have both the *blood* and *body* regulated to the higheft degree of purity and perfection; fuch fyftem of information may be readily acquired by proper attention to the neceffary inculcation and judicious obfervation, previous to the commencement of the feafon. This fact, founded upon the criterion of experience, naturally leads us into an enquiry what thofe preparations are, and the neceffity for their introduction: thefe we fhall confequently advert to, but not without an oblique remembrance of, and reference to, thofe Cynical cavillifts who (apprehending no dan-

ger

ger till they feel it) fet *phyfic at defiance* ; and never fubmit to acknowledge its utility, till the total lofs of one horfe and the irreparable injury to another, demonftrate the abfurdity of their ill-founded objections ; compulfively adding them in rotation to the annually en-creafing lift of converts to a rational fyfte-matic mode of ftabularian improvement.

Such obftinate non-compliance with the juftified dictates of fafety refulting from ex-perience, can arife only from a total want of thought, or knowledge of the animal econo-my ; by which every *fecretion, evacuation,* motion and labour is regulated, or action con-trouled. From the concurring force of this reflection, let every SPORTSMAN whofe mind is at all open to the rays of refinement, (and who has not, like TONY LUMPKIN, imbibed his entire ftock of penetration from the apron-ftring of a Mrs. *Hardcaftle,* conducting his whole affairs by " the rule of Thumb,") confider the abfolute neceffity of beftowing fome little occafional attention to the indica-tions of NATURE ; the direct procefs of *ali-ment* and *digeftion,* with its fubfequent fource of *nutrition* ; enabling himfelf to afcertain (at leaft with fome degree of precifion) the ftate

U 3 of

of his own horfes in ficknefs or health ; to difcover their neceffities, and prefcribe the remedies, without a degrading dependence upon the accumulated ignorance and affected confequence of every illiterate *groom, offler,* or *ftable boy* ; who, it is univerfally known, proudly poffefs obfolete receipts for every poffible difeafe to which the horfe is liable, (without its containing perhaps one applicable ingredient) and will valiantly vouch for the INFALLIBILITY OF ITS VIRTUES, though it is ten to one he is totally unacquainted with the articles of which it is compofed, and ftill more probably has not ability to read the *very farrago* he fo confidently recommends.

This evil has originally arifen, and been encreafed in its growth by too implicit, or rather too indolent, a fubmiffion of mafters in general, to the indifcreet (not to add *fometimes infernal*) and ridiculous propofitions of thefe people, upon whofe deftructive affectation of knowledge I have already fo repeatedly expatiated under different heads ; but am by practical obfervations, as often brought to a renewal of the fubject, to place every gentleman

tleman or fportfman on his guard againft
their inceffant obtrufions of medical judgment ; having within the laft few days heard
a moft illiterate puppy of the clafs defcribed,
propofe the infinuation of *lump fugar* for a
defect IN THE EYE, without a fingle reafon
to affign for the fupport of his recommendation, but that " it was like enough to do it
good."

This idea is too fublime and expanded for
a fingle remark in animadverfion ; but furely
every proprietor of horfes muft find it greatly
conducive to a promotion of his own eafe
and intereft, if he would condefcend to pay
fuch attention to this fubject, as might undoubtedly contribute a proportion of confidence to his additional knowledge ; and totally exculpate him from the mortifying predicament of appealing to the barren capacity
of his fervant in a MATTER OF MAGNI-
TUDE, whofe underftanding or inftructions
he would not fubmit to *confult*, or even condefcend to *hear*, upon much more inferior
occafions.

There has always exifted a diverfity of
U 4 opinions

opinions refpecting the propriety of purging horfes previous to the commencement of the hunting feafon; and this, as I have before hinted, has been one of the long ftanding difhes of contention between the *rights and the wrongs* ; it will be therefore expected (by thofe impartial inveftigators who are not blinded by invincible prejudice, but open to the conviction arifing from reafon) that fomething fhould now be advanced to juftify or condemn, what from not profeffionally underftanding the operative procefs of, or its effects upon the frame, has hitherto fufpended their opinions, not knowing *with juftice* which method to avoid, which to purfue.

That the matter may, however, be brought nearer the criterion of decifion, by being more clearly explained ; I fhall endeavour (without indulging a wifh to attract unneceffarily the attention of any reader from what he may conceive an object of greater importance) to convey fuch defcription of its neceffity, its operation upon the blood, and falutary effects upon the conftitution ; as I am induced to believe will prevent the *confiftency* of PURGING being longer a matter of controverfy;

controverfy ; but that upon certain and proper
occafions, it will become univerfally adopted
under the conditional regulations fo accurately explained in our former volume of this
work. Thofe inftructions, however, appertaining more particularly to the compofition
of various forms, the act of adminiftration,
and the mode of action upon the inteftinal
contents ; we advert now to the more remote
confideration of its *operative effects* upon the
ENTIRE SYSTEM, in juftification of its
adoption previous to the annual exertions of
violence, that fo evidently encreafe the velocity of the blood.

It may be remembered, that in my former
volume, under inftructions for getting horfes
into *condition*, I have recommended the operation of bleeding in a few days after being
taken from grafs ; by faying, " a proportion
may be taken away, according to the fize,
ftate, ftrength, and temperament of the horfe,
with due attention to the flefh he may have
gained, or the impurities he may have imbibed with his pafture." This paffage is fo
truly expreffive, and conveys to the mind fo
much in fo fhort a manner, that I have been
induced

induced to repeat the very words; as directly conducive to the fupport of an affertion frequently brought forward, " the great advantage of difcovering the true ftate of the blood."

The reafons are not only exceedingly obvious, but have been in their refpective parts fo minutely explained, that there is barely room to urge the propriety and enforce the utility of what ought to be laid down as the almoft fundamental rule of *phyfical* rectification; and, however abftrufe fuch reafoning may appear to the unfcientific and fuperficial part of the Vulcanian fraternity, denominated FARRIERS; I hefitate not a moment to affirm, there are very many cafes, in which I fhould be profeffionally induced to regulate the PHYSIC in both *quantity* and *quality,* by appearances accurately drawn from the ftate of the blood only.

What! (fays the furprifed and divided reader) when his Majefty's Farrier for Scotland has confidently affured us, and under the honourable fanction of royal appointment,

7

ment, that no difcovery can be made from the blood in any ftate whatever! That " blood drawn from a horfe who is evidently difordered, will fometimes have the fame appearance when cold, as that drawn from a horfe in health." And, *hey prefto!* VICE VERSA! " On the other hand, blood drawn from a horfe in health, will fometimes have all the appearance of that drawn from one labouring under the moft dangerous difeafe." All this Mr. Clarke may " *moft potently believe,*" yet " I hold it wrong to have it thus fet down ;" it bears fo great an affinity to the *ambiguous putting off* of HAMLET to his inquifitive companions, when he ferioufly affures them,

" There's ne'er a villain dwelling in all Denmark,
" But he's an arrant knave."

However, that jarring opinions may be the more eafily reconciled, I will venture to conclude for this very judicious and enlightened writer, that he intended to have *faid,* or wifhed it to be *underftood* ; That the cafes in which the blood of *difeafed horfes* bore the appearance of *horfes in health*.

health, were thofe very few in which the ftate of the blood is not fymptomatically affected by the difeafe; as *flatulent* or *inflammatory cholic*, *ftrangury*, and *worms*. But the better to exculpate myfelf from the accufation or even unjuft fufpicion of indulging the fhadow of inclination to arraign the authority, or fport with the judgment I fo very much refpect; let us charitably adopt AN ALTERNATIVE, and fuppofe, what is not only *poffible* but *probable*, that as the horfes in that country differ fo very materially from ours, (as thofe can teftify who have vifited the fpot, and recollect their appearance) why may not the *fluids* partake of the contraft? and their properties not being fo eafily or accurately analized as in the more fertile regions of the fouth; the line of diftinction we may naturally conclude is circumfcribed by the vermicular boundary of the *Tweed*, conftituting other diverfities of equal admiration.

From this digreffion, fo unavoidably neceffary to juftify my former recommenda-tion of BLEEDING, under proper reftrictions, we return to the confideration of

PURGING;

PURGING; upon the very falutary and judicious interpofition of which, I have already given my decided opinion as to its general utility, though I do not. mean to affert myfelf an advocate for its *indifcriminate* adminiftration, without due deference to the *caufe* and *condition* of the fubject. I wifh by no means to be confidered an invariable friend to unneceffary evacuations; perfectly convinced they are only *abfolutely* requifite, under the weight of injudicious accumulation. I therefore beg no mifconftruction may be put upon the thefis I advance, which is, that EVACUATIONS become not only *proper* but *indifpenfible*, when a horfe is SO MUCH ABOVE HIM-SELF in condition, that he evidently difplays the advancing progrefs and ill effects of repletion (arifing from full feed and irregular exercife) in the variety of ways fo repeatedly defcribed; not only under other heads in this, but different parts of the former volume, where the ftate of the blood neceffarily became the fubject of difquifition.

From what has been fo fully advanced
upon

upon the article of nutrition, circulation, evacuation, and exercise, it must be perfectly and systematically clear to every comprehension; that a horse too plethoric in habit, too much loaded with flesh, too viscid in the state of his blood, or too little accustomed to exercise, can never be brought into such strong exertions as the chace, without a very great probability of exciting inflammation, that may terminate in different degrees of disease, danger, and disquietude. Admitting therefore its indispensible necessity with horses of the above description, it must be taken into the aggregate; that although great inconveniencies and distressing circumstances may *possibly* arise, from the want of precaution in not bringing such preventatives into use, where the frame is replete with impurities; it can by no means follow that by the omission, with horses in any *tolerable condition,* the probable consequence becomes inevitable.

To draw the line of distinction between subjects rendering it a matter of necessity *with one,* or prudence and prevention only

only with *another*; it must be candidly acknowledged, that instances frequently occur, where horses perfectly clean, healthy, and without visible cause to suspect foulness in the body, or impurity in the blood, have by proper attention to stable management, good feeding, and regular exercise, been brought into the field in no degraded condition, and gone through the season with a moderate degree of perfection. Though this should not be attempted till an attentive observation to the state of the *coat*, *eyes*, *legs*, *heels*, the *wind* in brushing gallops, and the quality or appearance of the perspirative matter in the act of transpiration, may justify a reliance upon the faith of experiments; as latent impurities, or gross viscidities may remain dormant in the constitution, till roused into action by effects too numerous and extensive to admit of reiterated explanation, without deviating too largely from the subject it is our present purpose to pursue.

Having introduced remarks that were unavoidable, to demonstrate the consistency of carrying off such superflux as may constitute ftitute a preternatural weight upon the 'animal œconomy, by encumbering the infinity of finer veffels fo exquifitely concerned in fecretion and circulation, throwing the more noble parts of the machine into diforder; we proceed to explain the operative procefs and effects of CATHARTIC EVACUANTS upon the general fyftem; by which phyfical operation, nature becomes gradually relieved from the plethoric burthen of repletion, affecting even the moft diftant parts of the extremities, by means fo univerfally known and repeatedly defcribed.

PURGING, in its common and fuperficial acceptation with the unenlightened multitude, is confidered merely as a ready and convenient mode of expelling a load of accumulated contents from the ftomach, or excrements from the inteftines; without a relative confideration, or fingle idea of its more remote and falutary influence upon thofe parts of the frame, that are in general eftimation fuppofed to be very little concerned in the operation or its effects.

To elucidate this matter, and render it perfectly comprehenſible, (with as little reference as poſſible to abſtruſe reaſoning or anatomical diſquiſition) let it be underſtood, that the internal coat of the ſtomach is ſo plentifully portioned with branches from the nervous ſyſtem, that it may with great propriety be termed the joint ſeat of irritability ; for excluſive of the acting ſtimulus of the cathartic medicines upon the extreme ſenſibility of the nerves, ſo innumerably diſperſed in their different ramifications, they act alſo by irritation upon the mouths of the *lacteals* and *lymphatics*, exciting a continued and proportional emiſſion of their contents into the inteſtinal canal, ſo long as the ſtimulative properties of the medicine may have power to act ; during which ſuch abſorption of LYMPH, and regurgitation of CHYLE, intermixes with, and is carried off by the excrements.

By this conſtant *ſtimulus* upon the exquiſite ſenſibility of the ſtomach and inteſtines, the vermicular motion is not only excited to a more frequent diſcharge of its contents, but its continued irritation of the vaſcular ſyſtem

pro-

produces an increafed fecretion of *lymph* and *chyle*, which in the procefs of abforption and contribution to the excrementitious expulfion, is proportionally fupplied (or the veffels replenifhed) from even the moft diftant part of the extremities ; which evidently accounts for the vifible advantages arifing from a courfe of phyfic, when a horfe labours under the inconveniencies refulting from repletion ; and is faid, in the *Vulcanian phrafeology*, to have the HUMOURS fallen into the legs, or fixed upon any particular part of the frame.

Thus much is introduced to render perfectly clear, what I term the mechanical procefs of purgation ; by ftrictly attending to which it will evidently appear, that the weaker a cathartic is in its property, the lefs it will affect the fluids fufpended in different parts of the frame ; for its *firft ftimulus* acting upon the nervous fyftem as the *moft irritable*, the lymphatics and lacteals become only the fecondary feat of provocation, and are proportionally acted upon as the PHYSIC is increafed in its power of ftimulation.

From this very neceffary remark, I mean to infer,

infer, and wish it to be generally and incontrovertibly understood and held in remembrance, that a very moderate dose of physic will act in a great degree upon the irritability of the stomach and intestines *only*, exciting a discharge of their contents, as before described ; while its increased strength will, by its *additional stimulus* upon and persevering irritation of the finer vessels, excite their regurgitative contribution to the general evacuation, so long as the irritating properties of the cathartic shall retain the power of acting upon the vascular system ; which differing so very much in different subjects, requires proper discrimination in the composition of purging medicines, consequently, should always be carefully adapted to the state, constitution, and bodily strength of the horse.

This naturally leads us to an enquiry of the different degrees of PHYSIC, as most applicable to the various occasions for which they are brought into use. It evidently appears by the above investigation, that the *milder cathartics* act superficially, merely to discharge the contents of the intestinal ca-

nal ;

nal ; and are therefore calculated as preventatives to the *poffible* inconveniencies of impending repletion ; prefervatives of health, or
neceffary preludes to the completion of PER-
FECT CONDITION.

The fame elucidation likewife demon-
ftrates the confiftency of increafing the proportions, or enlarging the dofes, when more
diftant fervices are expected by calling the
remote powers into action, for the purpofes
fo particularly explained ; for inftance, in
great repletion of the veffels, fulnefs of the
carcafe, heavinefs of the head and eyes,
fwelling and tenfion of the legs, and fuch
other caufes as will be hereafter explained.
Gentle cathartics, acting merely as obfervable
laxatives, can never be expected to reach the
feat of thefe complaints ; fuch BRISK PURGES
only can be adopted with propriety, as will,
by their continued ftimulus, come into contact with, and additionally act upon, the very
interftices of the ftomach and inteftines, after
the excrementitious fuperflux is thrown off;
exciting by fuch means, the lymphatics and
lacteals to *difgorge* fome portion of their
extra contents, (diftinguifhed from time immemorial

memorial by the appellation of HUMOURS) to be ultimately carried off with the remaining efforts of inteftinal expulfion.

If any farther explanation can be at all required, to render this procefs more intelligible to the dulleft comprehenfions, I muft beg permiffion to recommend fuch Reader to a retrofpective recollection of his own fenfations towards the concluding operation of an emetic, or cathartic ; when I believe it will immediately occur to his remembrance, that the irritation of the veffels was much more fevere and effectual, (proved by the repeated ftrainings) than in the preceding difcharges when the contents were expelled with much greater eafe to the patient, though lefs efficacy upon the frame.

As I have juft hinted, there are other diforders, or rather *advanced ftages*, of thofe laft defcribed, (and for which " brifk purges" are recommended,) that require a ftill more peculiar mode of counter-action ; as horfes fubject to, or labouring under, inveterate *cracks* in the heels ; oozing indications of, or palpable greafe ; cutaneous *eruptions* ; vaf

X 3

cular

cular *knots*, or *tubercles*, the evident effects of plenitude; *worms*, or fluctuating pains in the limbs, occafioning alternate *lamenefs* in one part or another. In all which cafes, it is to be obferved, horfes fhould never have their exercife or labour increafed, to the leaft degree of violent exertion; without firft undergoing EVACUATIONS of fuch kind, as become immediately applicable to the cafe in queftion.

For my own part, I feel myfelf powerfully influenced to recommend the early adminiftration of *mercurial purges*, accurately proportioned to the ftate of the fubject and prevalence or duration of difeafe; and this upon the experimental bafis of minute attention to their fingular effects upon the conftitutions of horfes, in a variety of inftances that perfectly juftify me in communicating ESTABLISHED PROOFS of their fuperior excellence, not only in the different cafes juft recited, but in many others, that it would be foreign to our prefent purpofe to enumerate.

To prevent a perpetual obtrufion of technical

nical myftery, or medical difquifition, by enlarging upon the means of the mercurial particles entering into contact with the blood; its power of attenuation, gradual diffolution of the fluids and gentle ftimulation of the folids, (which muft at all times hang heavy upon the mind of the unfcientific enquirer); we muft let our abbreviated allufion fuffice, as a more fatisfactory mode of intelligent information, than a tedious chain of phyfical definition, that it may be thought has been already introduced by much too often.

In this tribute to the almoft incredible effects derived from the judicious and falutary interpofition of MERCURIAL CATHARTICS, I beg to difclaim every idea of patronizing fuch compofitions, prepared from the prefcriptive fcraps of antiquity, in the poffeffion of every *bellows blower* in the kingdom; not more in refpect to the probable difproportion and certain danger of their ingredients, than the abfurd, improper, and indifcriminate mode of introduction. Of thefe preparations, as of the various noftrums and quack medicines of the prefent day, I hold

the

the fame uniform and invariable opinion ; that the public are eternally peftered with innumerable advertifements, announcing the *miraculous cures*, (NATURE HAS PERFORMED) but not a fingle word of the many thoufands fuch medicines have deftroyed : So true it is, *" dead men tell no tales."*

Having gone through what I conceive a duty incumbent, refpecting the operation of phyfic and its effects upon the frame, to elucidate, as much as circumftances would admit, a fubject that has been hitherto confidered as fufficient matter to juftify and fupport a contrariety of opinions ; I muft, after giving it fuch profeffional explanation as my flender abilities were adequate to, fubmit the propriety of the practice, *under conditional regulations,* to the decifion of thofe who may do me the honour of minutely inveftigating, what has been neceffarily advanced for general confideration : Begging permiffion to obferve, that particular inftructions for the management of horfes under the operation of PHYSIC, may be found in the former volume under that head ; the prefent pages having been dedicated entirely to the operative

rative procefs and its effects upon the conftitution, for the purpofe of *univerfal* or rather
common comprehenfion.

That tafk having been at length performed,
we take leave of the dry and unentertaining ftudy of medical abftrufity, and proceed
to fuch part of our plan as will prove more
entertaining and acceptable to thofe, who
may condefcend to confult us for either
amufement or information. I have promifed
under the prefent head, rules for the felection of HUNTERS, and fome ufeful hints for
their management in the ftable and chace.
In refpect to the former, fuch defcriptive
parts as conftitute uniformity and the points
of perfection, will be found fo accurately
delineated in the early pages of our former
volume, that its repetition would bear too
much the appearance of literary impofition;
from which accufation, it has been our earneft endeavour, in every page, to ftand clearly
exculpated.

Upon the fubject of felection there can
therefore be but little to introduce beyond
the neceffity of adhering in choice, as much
as

as poffible to thofe that are *well-bred*, or, in other words, fuch as come the neareft in pedigree, fymmetry, fafhion, and apparent ftrength to thofe in conftant ufe for the turf, bearing the denomination and figure of BLOOD HORSES, as moft adequate in fpeed and durability (*termed bottom*) to long and fevere chaces with fleet hounds or in deep countries; under which, horfes of an inferior defcription fo frequently fink for want of that conftitutional ftamina or inherent fortitude, that horfes of high pedigrees are fo eminently known to poffefs.

From this eftablifhed and incontrovertible fact, we are naturally induced to introduce a few oblique remarks upon the very neceffary qualification of " BONE ;" fo fafhionably and eternally echoed and tranfmitted (in equeftrian infpection) from one affected puppy to another, that they feem to have anticipated, or rather premeditated, the inexpreffible pleafure of difcovering what they call " *a want of bone*" in the horfes of *others*, that they unluckily feldom or ever perceive in *their own*. Thefe curious obfervers, (mere pretenders to judgment) never condefcend to

investigate

investigate caufes or effects, farther than as at firft fight they affect the fuperficies of their very fhallow comprehenfion; from whence arifes the prevalent reflection upon the *want of bone*, fo exceedingly common, and fo frequently *ill-founded*, that at the time of examination, the fubject fo difparaged is fometimes loaded like a cart horfe. From this total ignorance of the anatomical conformation, has originated the erroneous conjecture of fixing the bafis of ftrength in the bony ftructure *only*, without a contingent reference or relative confideration to the mufcular appendages, that, in fact, conftitute the very main fpring of ftrength and action.

We are not at all difinclined to admit that the greater the fulcrum or mechanical centre of fupport, the more powerful fhould be the component parts to conftitute the accumulation of ftrength; though this, like many other rules fuppofed to be general, is liable to frequent exception. Of this there are diftinct proofs among the different degrees of horfes, in the particular purpofes for which they are bred, or afterwards become

appro-

appropriate to; for inftance, horfes bred with ftrength for _draft_, or with fpeed for the _chace_, are fo directly oppofite in fome part of their _fhape_, and the whole of their _requifites_, that what conftitutes perfections for the one, difplays an abfolute deficiency for the other.

Hence arifes the inconfiftency of bringing crofs-bred heavy horfes into the chace, where their own weight, and want of action, lay the foundation of their deficiency; for in hard or long running they become inevitably exhaufted, and frequently fall victims to the imprudent perfeverance of their riders. Thofe juvenile or inattentive fportfmen, whofe experience has been exceedingly limited, or obfervations confined, may not yet be perfectly convinced that BLOOD HORSES (notwithftanding the popular clamour of their deficiency in bone) will exceed in _fpeed, ftrength,_ and _bottom_, whatever horfes of an oppofite defcription may be brought into the field; and of this fact I am fo exceedingly well convinced by experimental obfervation and unremitting attention, that in a long chace

with

with fleet hounds, running *breaſt high*, and *acroſs a country*, nothing but horſes three parts or thorough bred can ever lay by the ſide of them.

In addition alſo to this truth, let us encounter the full force of another notion equally ridiculous, and well calculated for thoſe who hunt in *theory*, and enjoy the chace upon *paper*; of " a blood horſe not having bone and ſtrength ſufficient to cover *a deep and dirty country*;" when every ſportſman of experience, who has made the trial impartially, will join with me in the aſſertion, that horſes of that deſcription abſolutely poſſeſs the ſtrength (in their great power of action and pliability) to paſs over ſuch country, with very ſlight impreſſion and no great labour; when it is a matter not to be controverted, that a ſtrong heavy horſe, not only ſinks deep with his own weight at every ſtroke, but extricates himſelf with the utmoſt difficulty, leaving his rider in the pleaſing predicament of ſoon enquiring " which way the hounds are gone?" with the greater gratification of poſſeſſing a horſe

of

of *bone and strength* sufficient to carry him
" AFTER *any pack of hounds in the kingdom."* Having before bid adieu to medical
myftery and anatomical defcription, we do
not mean to renew the fubject by a comparative detail of mufcles and tendons, with
their appertaining confiderations; but leave
every reader to make up his own mind upon
the qualifications and kind of horfe moft applicable to his idea of the chace, and intention of riding with or *after* the hounds;
proceeding to a communication of fuch remarks as, properly attended to, may be productive of their different degrees of utility.

It may be remembered, that the different
fubjects of PHYSIC, EXERCISE, and CON-
DITION have all been feparately confidered,
and their advantages accurately explained;
as may be perceived by application to the
index of either volume for information upon
any particular head. We now confequently
arrive at the commencement of the hunting
feafon, when, meeting in the field, every
countenance betrays a heart elate with the
general effufion of joy that is to enfue. Previous to farther animadverfion upon which,

it

it becomes neceffary to remark, that the extreme degree of perfection, and high condition I have hitherto recommended, and allude to in my future inftructions for ftable management, are by no means intended to be generally extended to horfes in common ufe with HARRIERS; whofe offices of fervice are fo exceedingly different to the very ftrong and fevere chaces with STAG or FOX, that they may naturally be underftood to be always fufficiently prepared with a very inferior treatment.

Left fuch gentlemen, who from fituation, inclination, advanced age, or bodily debilitation, are attached to the frigidity of HARE HUNTING, fhould feel the dignity of *their pack,* and the *fplendor of their retinue,* degraded by what they may erroneoufly conceive an oblique infinuation of contempt; I muft beg to fubmit to the criterion of their own decifion, the almoft incredible difference between the exertions and duration of the two. Horfes that become the neceffary appendage to *harriers,* undergo fuch fudden changes in their fport, not more in the frequent dull and tedious attendance upon the hounds
when

6

when trailing to find in the cold and chilling dreary fog of a fevere winter's morning;
than the alternate contrasts in the chace,
arising from those checks in " *heading, turning, doubling,* and *squatting,*" that conftitute firft a burft to promote perspiration, then
a "*fault*" to fupprefs it.

This is fo very oppofite to the violent and
continued exertions of a chace with either
STAG or FOX, in the prefent improved
breed and fleetnefs of hounds; that I only
mean to convey an idea of the probable
hazard of having a horfe kept in too high a
ftile for a chace fo fubject to fluctuation in
the different degrees of *heat* and *cold,* that a
horfe. in perfect condition muft have great
good fortune, or an excellent conftitution, not to feel the ill effects of long attendance upon HARRIERS, at leaft in thofe
countries where the fcarcity of game admits of much loft time between *killing* and
finding. For my own part, however repugnant the opinion may prove to one
clafs of fportfmen; I feel myfelf juftified in
declaring, no confideration whatever fhould
influence me to dance attendance upon har-

4   riers,

riers, with a horse of great value and tolerable perfection, unless a certainty of expeditiously finding, and inceffant running, might induce me to *exercife a horfe* on the intermediate days, as a prelude to the chace with either of the other two.

Confidering, therefore, the management we allude to, as appertaining more particularly to horfes of high qualifications, we advert, as before mentioned, to the commencement of the feafon; when, at the place of meeting, every fportfman feels eager for the fport and replete with emulation. That we may omit no inftruction or advice, however minute, that can at all contribute to the pleafure or fafety of the chace : let it be held in remembrance, the frame (or rather the ftomach) fhould never be loaded when entering into immediate action. The portions of hay and water fhould be adminiftered with a very fparing hand, for the laft twelve or fixteen hours preceding the chace; to which end hay fhould be reftricted in quantity more on that night than any other, his evening and morning feeds of corn being increafed in

proportion to the deficiency in the other
part of his aliment. On the morning of
hunting he fhould be dreffed and fed early ;
having his head ftrapped up till faddled for
the field, to prevent (if a coarfe feeding horfe)
his making the clean ftraw a neceffary fubftitute for the artificial fcarcity of hay.

The day preceding which, every judicious
or experienced fportfman arranges all his affairs, to prevent the leaft probability of delay,
difappointment, or interruption to his fport;
by accurately afcertaining the adequate ftate
of his horfe and the fafety of his apparatus.
He defcends to an attentive furvey of the feet
and the *clinches* of the *fhoes* ; thereby avoiding the diftreffing dilemma of compulfively
exploring a SMITH'S SHOP, in a ftrange
country, during the heat and happinefs of
the *chace*, by the inexpreffible mortification
of *cafting a fhoe*: A circumftance that will
feldom or never happen under the occafional
infpection of the fmith, who will moft certainly never forget the PROPER or accuftomed time of examination ; provided he is
retained upon the principle of *mutual conve-*
nience,

nience, fo particularly explained in 138 and the following pages.

Proper attention fhould follow to the form of the faddle and the ftate of its ftuffing, to prevent even the poffibility of the tree coming into injurious contact with the *wither;* or the probability of *warbles,* by the indentation or friction of the girth buckles, in a long or fevere chace. The girth web for hunting fhould be what is termed " fpring web" in preference, for the advantage of its additional elafticity; the harfh, tight wove web, very frequently occafioning a laceration of the integument, known by the name of " *bowel galled.*" If due refpect was alfo paid to the probable durability of the *ftirrup leathers,* it might certainly render fuperfluous the paltry difplay of a NEW BELT round the body of A GENTLEMAN, indicating a fafe refource for a *broken leather;* a piece of equeftrian oftentation never practifed by fportfmen of eftablifhed reputation, who are univerfally known to be too-fubftantially provided, in fo material a part of their equipments, to ftand the moft diftant chance of an accident, that would not only retard their

Y 2   progrefs,

progress, but inevitably *throw them out*, before they could repair their lofs, if the hounds were then crossing a country.

If horses have not six or eight miles to the hounds on the morning of hunting, they should be walked at least an hour, or hour and half, before they appear at the place of meeting; the consistency of their having sufficient time to unload the frame by frequency of evacuation, has been so fully explained under the article of exercise, and its palpable utility must be so forcibly striking to every person at all convinced of its effects, that it cannot possibly require any additional elucidation.

Supposing ourselves arrived at that unsullied seat of unanimity the place appointed, whether throwing into covert for a FOX, or turning out the DEER; every sportsman will acknowledge it may be justly deemed the critical moment, when the powers of exhilaration nearly exceed the limits of prescription, and we " most wonder how our reason holds." This is the crisis that too frequently deprives the juvenile rider (in

8   his

his initiation) of the degree of prudence fo exceedingly neceffary in the early part of the chace ; particularly at the beginning of the feafon, when they are fo little inured to exertions of violence and fatigue. The *firft burft*, with either DEER or FOX, is generally fevere, and not unfrequently of long duration, in which too much tendernefs cannot be beftowed upon the very fountainhead of your pleafure ; from whofe perfections and perfeverance only, you can derive your enjoyment of the chace. It is therefore perfectly right to have it ever in remembrance, that the more moderately a horfe is exerted in the early part of the day, the greater probability you infure of feeing the end of it ; with the pleafing confolation of eafe to your horfe, and no bad compliment to your own reputation ; for it is a well known fact, that there are hundreds in a feafon, who from an impatient defire and eager impetuofity to fee too much of the *beginning*, feldom or never know much of the *conclufion*, promoting by indifcretion the very means of their mortification and difgrace.

Y 3

Moderation

Moderation in the chace, and steady attention to the leading hounds, will constantly
prevent confiderable difficulty to the rider,
as well as the horfe : This is a matter,
however, more " devoutly to be wifhed,"
than at all to be expected. It is equally
natural to conclude, that moft of thofe adherents attached to and enjoying the chace,
would regulate the *fpeed* of their horfes
by the depth of the ground they go over;
obfervation daily convinces us it is not fo,
and that there are very numerous exceptions to fuch neceffary and laudable circumfpection.

Experience conftantly affords us demonftrative proof, that nothing fo much exhaufts the bodily ftrength, reduces the
fpeed, and exhaufts the wind, as ftrong and
repeated leaps *in any,* but particularly *in
deep countries :* This reflection ought furely
to convince young or unthinking riders,
that fuperfluous leaps, and unneceffary difficulties, fhould never be boaftingly encountered, to difplay an affectation of equeftrian
courage, or pragmatic confequence; for
they immediately (in the mind of every prudent

dent and humane obferver) appear fo many incontrovertible proofs of his ignorance or indifcretion. Thefe HEROES ON HORSEBACK require to be emphatically informed, that fuch voluntary acts of oppreffion invariably operate to the prejudice of the performer, however he may be fanctioned by fituation or favoured by fortune, proving unluckily abortive of the original defign; for what is fo evidently intended to create admiration, is as certainly productive of indifference and contempt.

Another act of folly and indifcretion is equally calculated to excite the difguft and indignation of every eftablifhed fportfman in the field; that ridiculous vanity of try- ing the fpeed and oppreffing the fpirit of your horfe, in *racing* with every fympa- thetic competitor; and it would be very extraordinary in fo numerous a company, if *one fool* was long deprived the pleafure of finding *a companion*. At the conclufion of the chace, whether the death of a FOX or the taking of the DEER, numerous temptations prefent themfelves to the young and inexperienced fportfman, even in the

Y 4 infancy

infancy of his initiation ; while encountering the various propofitions of the company,
fufpended in opinion between the prevalence
of inclination and power of confiftency.

Previous to the remarks I proceed to make,
it is not inapplicable to introduce one obfervation relative to a termination of the diftinct
chaces I have juft had occafion to mention ;
for though the former muft be candidly
acknowledged proportionally fevere in its
courfe, it is by no means comparative in its
duration. His MAJESTY's *Red Deer*, under
the acknowledged excellence of their prefent
eftablifhment, exceed in the length of their
runs all former remembrance, and almoft every
conception of thofe unacquainted with the fubject ; from *three* to *four* hours may be candidly
confidered the average of each chace, with
deer in high condition ; at the conclufion of
which, it is no uncommon circumftance to
be *twenty, five and twenty,* or *thirty* miles
from home, or the place of turning out.

This is the period when every imprudent
or impatient rider fhould exert his judgment
to difcover the ftate of his horfe and regulate
his

his proceedings accordingly ; horſes are never ſo perfectly at eaſe as in their *own ſtables,* which they ſhould attain with all poſſible convenience. There are numbers who (without at all adverting to the length of the chace, or their diſtance from home,) may be conſtantly obſerved eagerly enquiring the *neareſt way* to the firſt houſe of public accommodation, making what converts they can by example ; where, without a reference to contingencies, horſes in ſuch ſtate are raſhly conſigned to the *unſullied care* and *inceſſant attention* of the IMMACULATE OSTLER, (if the premiſes are enabled to produce one) when they are *ordered* to be " well cleaned," " properly fed," and " ſufficiently watered." This important truſt (for ſuch it certainly is when thoroughly inveſtigated) is thus delegated to an inferior power, that is perhaps in five minutes unavoidably compelled to abandon it, and accept of a *ſecond* or *third,* which may be no more in his power to execute. Thus the commiſſion is going on, while the *happy inadvertent* owners are gratifying their appetites and drowning their cares in all the luxuries of the manſion ; indulging their vanity in a recital of their perſonal exploits,

ploits, and an alternate defcription of the difficulties they had furmounted in the feve- rities of the chace.

To thofe in the laudable habits of a dif- ferent practice, animadverfion upon the danger becomes fuperfluous; but as there are thofe, who it is impoffible to convince of their errors, till repentance comes too late, it may prove no unfeafonable admonition to declare, from this kind of treatment only, I have been a witnefs to *repeated inftances,* where the horfes have never been brought again out of the ftable, but in woeful pro- ceffion to the *Collar Makers,* who had pur- chafed their hides.

The ftripping of a horfe to drefs him in a comfortlefs ftable, with every pore of the frame relaxed to its utmoft extenfion, and the additional *happy introduction* of a pail of COLD WATER (as moft applicable to the convenience of the *oftler* or his *deputy*) has been the deftruction of more horfes in dif- ferent ways, than ever fuffered by the longeft and moft terrible runs when rode with dif- cretion. So much has been repeatedly in- troduced

troduced upon the repulsion of perspirative matter, from the surface to the different parts of the frame, that not a single line can be required in elucidation of so clear a part of the subject.

Steady and attentive observance has, years since, convinced me of the inconsistency of approaching a house of this kind in the general hurry and confusion, with any hope of obtaining the requisite attendance your horse may prove in need of; a diffident applicant may stand his hour unnoticed, and his gentle requests unanswered, while those fortunately possessed of unbounded confidence and fashionable effrontery may probably succeed in their applications. It is therefore much more commendable to pass gently on with your horse to a house whose present engagements are not so numerous, which may generally be found in a few miles of your way homeward; here you become so much the object of attention, that you almost obtain in anticipation what you could not before acquire by the most humble entreaty. This answers your purpose perhaps in another respect, as your horse will have become cool and proper for what

attention

attention you find it neceffary to beftow; for no horfe whatever, after a fevere run, fhould be placed in a ftable, or fuffered to ftand ftill, till the encreafed velofity of the blood and the confequent perfpiration had gradually fub-fided to its former temperance.

When your place of temporary conveni-ence is obtained, let be only thirty or forty minutes at moft, for the following purpofes of evacuation and nutrition: See that the ftable, and the ftall in that ftable, are made as near the warmth of your own as circum-ftances will permit; let the bridle be taken off, a handful of fweet hay thrown before him, the girths flackened, and the faddle *juft loofened* only from the back, to which it may adhere clofely by the long continued perfpi-ration; let a fheet (or fuch fubftitute as the place affords) be thrown over his hind quar-ters, and the litter be plentifully fpread under his belly, to excite a falutary difcharge of urine, (by this time much wanted) obferving that he ftales without difficulty, and difplays no figns of ftrangury; if fo, they muft be attended to in the manner defcribed in the former volume, fhould nature be tardy in her

own

own relief and the violence of fymptoms
increafe.

Procraftinate any wants of YOUR OWN,
and make up the deficiencies of the *day* in
the extra comforts of the *evening* ; this will
infure you the exquifite fenfation arifing
from an act of juftice and humanity. Depend upon no pompous inftructions for the
doubtful fupply of *warm water* neceffary to
your purpofe or intention : diveft yourfelf of
the rank folly of falfe confequence, and attend to the *immediate procuration* ; examine
its proper warmth, and be yourfelf the trufty
fuperintendant, unlefs the favours of fortune
and the fidelity of your fervant have luckily
placed you above the neceffity of perfonal
attendance. So foon as he has *ftaled*, let his
head be well rubbed with part of a foft hay
band, and thoroughly cleanfed with the brufh ;
draw his ears repeatedly through the hands,
all which will prove perfectly refrefhing.
The legs fhould be alfo well rubbed down
with double whifps, to prevent an obftruction
of the pores, or ftiffnefs from accumulated
dirt and perfpiration.

This

This done, let a moderate feed of the best corn your *local granary* affords, be thrown into the manger, and the door of the stable immediately closed.   Having thus conscientiously discharged the incumbent office of grateful protection; embrace the few minutes you have to spare in obtaining for yourself, what little refreshment nature stands in need of.   Let no inducement whatever from more unthinking companions, attract your attention from the state of your horse to the circulation of the bottle; if once you suffer your sober judgment to relax from what should be the invariable maxim of your perseverance, you know not where the indiscretion ends; one single step of deviation from the line of prudence and propriety, frequently introduces a thousand more to promote contrition.

Upon ample demonstration, that every horse, supported in a domestic stile, has as fervent an attachment to his own stall as his master to his own bed, and will most cheerfully encounter (if necessary) much additional fatigue to attain it; there is no doubt but it is highly commendable to bridle him

so

fo foon as his corn is finifhed, and take him gently home, provided the diftance is not *too great*, to prevent a comfort fo truly defirable to both the horfe and his rider. In this recommendation I feel myfelf perfectly juftified, not only upon the experimental advantage of frequently taking my horfe (in the way I have defcribed) upwards of twenty miles to his own ftall, which has been my invariable practice for more than twenty years, but the flattering gratification to obferve many of my friends as regularly follow the example.

No infectious folicitations, that fo conftantly feduce others to an *immediate* participation of *table comforts*, ever have the moft trifling weight in the fcale of MY DETERMINATION; dedicated entirely to the fafety of my horfe, no moment is unneceffarily wafted till he is " rewarded according to his deferts," and fafely lodged in his own ftable, beyond the probable reach of danger; where, upon his arrival, (whether after a long or fhort return from either a fevere or moderate chace) the mode of management is critically the fame; his legs and feet are not

only

only inftantly wafhed with warm water, but
in fo doing, the neceffary infpection made,
whether the moft trifling injuries have been
fuftained by over-reaches, ftubs, or in lace-
rations between hair and hoof; while this is
doing, a portion of hay is thrown before
him, and immediately after a pail of water,
flightly warm, to allay the violent thirft always occafioned by long and fevere chaces.
The ufual ceremony of dreffing, feeding,
oiling, ftopping, and other minutiæ of the
ftable is then gone through; too fyftematically and generally underftood to require a
fingle line in explanation.

· A perfeverance in this rigidity of ftable
difcipline and attention, unbiaffed by the
perfuafion or example of others, will always
infure you the fuperiority of *condition* in
the field; under the pleafing fenfation of
your horfe being at home, and completely
taken care of; when others, lefs con-
fiderate, or lefs humane, are commencing a
wretched journey of ten, fifteen, or twenty
miles in a dreary winter's evening; or
what is nearly upon a parallel of inconfiftency, permit them to remain in a ftrange
(and

(and perhaps cold and uncomfortable) ftable, to be badly fed and worfe looked after. But let it be either *one* or the *other*,
refulting confequences are much the fame ;
the porous fyftem is affected in a greater
or lefs degree, the coat becomes rough,
and unhealthy, bearing the appearance of
HIDE-BOUND, and the perfpirative matter
thus compulfively returned upon the circulation without abforption, muft evidently
foon appear to affect the eyes, lungs, or
glandular parts ; to the certain hazard of
blindnefs, afthma, broken wind, or fome one
of the contingent ills fo repeatedly alluded
to in various parts of this, as well as our
former volume.

Refpecting the article of FEEDING, various opinions are entertained, and perhaps
no fmall number of thofe regulated by
pecuniary confiderations ; it is, however, univerfally admitted, that HUNTERS require
a more extraordinary fupport than many
horfes of different denominations ; but the
particular reafons why *extra fupport* becomes fo immediately neceffary, is a matter but little underftood by thofe not much

fubject to abftrufe reafoning or remote conviction.

It has been repeatedly proved under the article of EXERCISE and its effects, that a want of action (when properly fupplied with food) overloads not only the frame with aliment, but the circulation with a fuperflux of nutrition; it muft therefore evidently appear, by parity of reafoning, that great and conftant exertions in the chace muft neceffarily exhauft the fluids by perfpiration, as the contents of the inteftines by evacuation; and unlefs the fyftem is fufficiently fupplied with nutritious, reftorative, and healthy aliment (the beft in its kind) for the due fupport of thefe frequent difcharges, impoverifhed blood, . lofs of flefh, dejected fpirit, and bodily debilitation, muft prove the inevitable confequence.

After the moft attentive obfervation I have been able to beftow for a number of years, cultivating an anxious defire to difcover the proper criterion of fupport and gratification for horfes of this defcription, who are fair feeders, and do their work well; I could never find that a lefs portion than feven pecks or two bufhels of corn, and two trufs (one hundred weight) of hay, per week, would keep them up to a proper degree of ftrength and appearance. This is the leaft quantity of either, that any horfe of my own confumes in the hunting feafon; which allowance will conftitute fome entertainment, in contraft with the weakly fubfiftence of thofe metropolitan ftables, fo particularly alluded to in page 199 of the work before us. In this calculation, the reader muft be informed, there is no conditional reference or allufion to horfes of *weak appetites*, that are off their food with every trifling exertion, or extra fatigue; they are by no means entitled to a ftall in the ftable of an experienced fportfman, who, when fuch accidentally fall into his poffeffion, will undoubtedly foon extricate himfelf from the incumbrance without the leaft neceffity for my recommendation.

WATER is fo equally and effentially requifite to the very exiftence of life, and performance of every function, that it be-

comes

comes entitled to a proper degree of confideration; but knowing (from the very
nature of the enquiry) how little attention
would be paid to a tedious and defultory
diffufion of matter, upon the different
kinds of water, their properties, the mineral particles they contain, the diftinct ftrata
through which they run and become impregnated as they pafs, with their *probable* or *poffible* effects upon the conftitutions of horfes, would lead us again into
a very extenfive and unentertaining field
of phyfical difquifition, that we wifh by
no means to renew, unlefs it could tend
to enlighten the fubject or improve the
judgment. In an attempt to fucceed effectually in either, BRACKEN muft be
eventually cited to juftify one affertion,
CLARKE to demonftrate another; the fum
total of all which, could amount only to
an accumulation of conjecture refpecting
ftone, gravel, and *ftrangury,* without any
thing being pofitively afcertained, by a catalogue of conditional fuppofitions, founded
upon the various properties of different
waters, according to the foils through
which

which they run, or from whence they are extracted.

In fact, such accurate investigation has been made by Mr. CLARKE of this subject, that it absolutely precludes every possibility of introducing a single line in addition, without the appearance of plagiarism ; but with due deference to his good intent, and true physical distinction, I cannot but conceive, that so general a description of the different kinds of water will afford but little satisfaction to those who are inevitably compelled to abide by the local properties of their own country, without the bare possibility of an alternative.

Taking this circumstance into consideration, I think it can be only necessary to take up the subject upon a general ground ; merely to introduce such few remarks upon the quantity and quality of water, as is evidently most applicable to the *state*, *condition*, and *purpose* of those horses whose situation, circumstances, or fluctuations of

weather,

weather, render their watering in the ftable a bufinefs totally unavoidable.

I have in different parts of my former volume, faid what then became applicable upon this fubject; but we now proceed a few fteps farther, in elucidation of any deficiency; and the more particularly as our remarks conftitute a link of continuity to the prefent chain of inftruction. It can never have efcaped the attention of the moft fuperficial obferver, what a wonderful change is almoft inftantaneoufly produced in the appearance and fenfations of a horfe, by a gratification of thirft in *well* or *pump* wa-ter, but more particularly if given in the ftable cold and in the winter feafon. In moft horfes a violent fhivering and ftaring of the coat immediately fucceed, and con-tinue more or lefs without intermiffion; thofe conftantly fupplied in this manner having always a coat nearly of two colours, (that is, one half ftanding on end, and the other part fmooth) difplaying a fcurfy dufty hue at the bottom, evidently the effect of a repeated collapfion of the porous fyftem and frequent obftruction of infenfible perfpiration.

To

To prevent, by every poſſible means, the hazard of ſuch inconvenience as muſt evidently enſue from treatment ſo highly improper; horſes ſhould invariably, when the ſeaſons and the ſtate of thoſe ſeaſons will permit, be watered abroad at either *pond* or *pool* of ſoft and well ſheltered water; as greatly preferable to the harſh and chilling frigidity of thoſe we have deſcribed. But even in this mode, a horſe ſhould never be permitted to glut himſelf to the leaſt degree of ſatiety; for having no regulator but appetite, no guide but inclination, they very frequently (under management of the inadvertent and inconſiderate) drink to an exceſs, occaſioning the moſt excruciating pain, and no trifling degree of danger and diſquietude. Six or ſeven quarts need never be exceeded to horſes of this claſs at one time, and that as regularly divided in reſpect to the *equal arrangement of time* as circumſtances will permit; to be repeated twice in twenty-four hours, at nearly the diſtance of *twelve* from each other, to avoid the frequent folly of having water *twice* in about *eight* hours, remaining SIXTEEN without.

Z 4

When

When the feverity of the weather, as *rain, froft,* or *fnow,* prevents horfes of this defcription from being watered in fuch way ; the only prudent alternative (to avoid every inconvenience) is to furnifh them *with foft water* -from fuch receptacles in the ftable, either in its natural ftate, or with the chill taken off, as the feafon and circumftances may require ; letting the fubject almoft immediately undergo a brifk brufhing over for a quarter of an hour or more, to enliven the circulation and prevent the difagreeable fenfations of rigor and the effect of obftructed perfpiration.

It now becomes neceffary we revert once more to the fubject of EXERCISE ; upon the utility of which, we have already enlarged, under its diftinct head, and from its numerous advantages and indifpenfible neceffity, cannot, in fact, be afraid of introducing too much ; it is the very fountain of health, appetite, and invigoration, without which, a horfe can never be adequate to the purpofe intended. Proper exercife for horfes, denominated HUNTERS, and appropriated to no other ufe, fhould be be almoſt *invariable* reſpecting manner, length of time and diſtance; though it muſt be univerſally known ſuch circumſtance becomes greatly dependent upon the ſeaſon of the year, the ſtate of the weather, the ſeverity of the preceding chace, and the condition of the horſe.

Under ſuch certain and unavoidable fluctuation, conditional inſtructions only can be admitted; ſubject as they muſt ever remain to the contingencies of inevitable diverſification. Horſes on the intervening days, during the *firſt* and *laſt* weeks of each ſeaſon, when the days are long and ſeaſons mild, ſhould be taken out twice a day; for inſtance, from eight to nine in the morning, and from four to five in the afternoon; giving them their proper portion of water at ſuch *pond* or *pool* of ſoft water as is moſt remarkable for its ſalubrious properties in the neighbourhood of reſidence. Let the exerciſe be moderate, and equally divided before and after the water; remembering, as already obſerved, to regulate the *length* and *ſtrength* of the exerciſe by the CONDITION of the horſe.

If

If he is of high spirit, and so much *above his work*, that he encreases in flesh, indicating the least display of foulness from repletion, let his exercise be proportionally extended; on the contrary, if the subject is of slender constitution, lax habit, light in the carcase, and weak appetite, the digestive powers must be consequently deficient, and proceedings regulated accordingly; becoming entirely dependent upon circumstances and judicious super-intendance.

In what I term the four centrical months of the hunting season, when the days are exceedingly short, and the weather severe; the mode of exercise must be varied, and rendered subservient to the changes that occur; taking them out at such times as may be found most convenient under difficulties that frequently arise. The rule, however, best adapted to general practice in favourable weather, is to let them have their exercise at once, and that in the middle of the day, between or from the hours of *eleven* to *one*; equally avoiding the chilling fogs of the morning, and damps of the evening: having it always in remembrance,

membrance, that when prevented (by the continuance of inceſſant rain, or deep fall of ſnow upon the ground) from taking them out at all, their dreſſings are increaſed, and patiently perſevered in, to enliven the circulation, promote the ſecretions and evacuations, as the only ſubſtitute for the more ſubſtantial advantage of regular exerciſe.

It is a caſe too frequently obſerved, and indeed almoſt generally known, that the horſes of Gentlemen are ſometimes unluckily ſubject, *in all weathers*, to a part of their exerciſe at the door of *an obſcure alehouſe*; for however hoſpitable may be the manſion of the maſter, ſtill the prevalence of " DAMNED CUSTOM" has rendered it ſo predominant, it is in a certain degree faſhionable with thoſe *faithful and truſty* ſervants, who, poſſeſſing neither innate principal nor perſonal gratitude, render the moſt valuable property of their employers dangerouſly ſubſervient to the paltry inconſiſtency and gratification of their own inclinations.

Having

Having omitted, upon the subject of diseased eyes, to introduce a matter of opinion that should have appeared with more propriety under the article of " SHOEING," and frequent ill usage of SMITHS; I am induced to submit it to consideration before I take leave of the subject before us. It is what I have ever thought a too unjustifiable and great exertion of strength, in the use and twist of *the twitch*, when a horse is put into that excruciating state of coercion for shoeing, or any other operation. In this extremity of pain and humiliation, the eyes are frequently observed agitated, even to the expulsion of tears, from the great irritability, and greater stimulation of the nervous system; this is so seldom regulated by the salutary interposition of *judgment*, *humanity*, and *discretion*, that I shall ever retain doubts, from the observations I have made, whether various defects in the eyes, or a paralytic state of the optic nerves, may not be very commonly produced by such means, when attributed to more remote causes.

R O A D

ROAD HORSES

ARE thofe in general performing the moft laborious work, and many of them enjoying the leaft accurate attention of any in the kingdom. It is in fact matter of furprife, that a part of the fpecies conftituting the very bafis and fupport of inland com- merce, the only means of expeditious travel- ling, and the advantages of general conveni- ence in bufinefs and pleafure, fhould be fo cruelly neglected, or indifferently treated, as may be plainly perceived (without the eyes of Argus) in almoft every *inn* and a va- riety of *private ftables* in every part of Eng- land.

Under this defcription come by much the greater part of all the horfes in conftant ufe; as it includes carriage horfes of every kind, roadfters and hacks, whether of GEN- TLEMEN, TRADESMEN, or TRAVELLERS (commonly called riders); all which con- ftitute an infinity, as well in the metropolis as every part of the country. A very great

9   proportion

proportion of thefe derive fo little fupport from the *ocular infpection* and *perfonal care* of their riders or drivers; that if the fecret interpofition of Providence did not influence a greater degree of affiftance in their favour, than thofe generally do who fhould be their protectors, more poverty and bodily deftruction muft inevitably enfue.

Rules for felecting horfes in purchafe are fo plainly inculcated in the early part of the former volume, that they claim no part of our prefent attention; management, with fuch hints only as appertain to the tuition of young and inexperienced travellers, will form the fum total of arrangement under this head. It would prove matter of aftonifhment to thofe not intimately acquainted with the general ftate, condition, and accommodation of horfes, what labour they execute, the incredible difficulties they furmount, the inceffant fatigue they patiently endure, and the little they fubfift on in the hands of hundreds, who feel no paffion but gain, no pride but infenfibility.

The horfes paffing under the denomination

tion of ROAD HORSES are fo exceedingly numerous of the different kinds, that a diftinct mode of treatment for each particular fort, would be extending the fubject to a length beyond the wifh and expectation of every reader. Such felection may therefore be made from the general advice, as the enquirer may find moft applicable to the ftate of his horfe and the purpofe of his appropriation; though the inftructions may be confidered as more confiftently adapted to faddle and light carriage horfes, than thofe employed in heavy machines, road waggons, and the inferior vehicles in conftant ufe.

Previous to farther embarkation upon that part of the fubject, it may not prove inapplicable to take an oblique furvey of thofe public receptacles known by the appellation of *inns*; originally intended and admirably calculated for the convenience and accommodation of travellers, but unfortunately, like many other inftitutions of general utility, perverted to the worft of purpofes; having become fo numerous (for the advantage of their LICENCED contribution to government) that they find it convenient to practife every degree

gree of impofition and every fpecies of adulteration, upon the plaufible plea of ftate neceffity and felf-prefervation.

Of thefe houfes there are in fact but **two**
diftinct kinds, that fall within the neceffary
circumfpection and remembrance of the traveller, for they are generally in the oppofite
extreme; the accommodations of one clafs
are *hofpitable, generous, humane,* and *confcientious;* the other, execrable to every excitement of INDIGNATION. While the former
are exerting every nerve to acquire fubfiftence
and obtain approbation, with honefty and
unfullied reputation; the latter are deriving
indifcriminate fupport by every degree of
DECEPTION without doors, and every fpecies of PECUNIARY oppreffion within. Servants, it is a maxim, foon acquire the *virtues*
or *vices* of their employers, if they indulge
a wifh to retain their fituations; and upon
the truth of that ancient adage, " birds of a
feather flock together," where you find the
wifh to pleafe predominant in the mafter or
miftrefs, you immediately obferve fympathetic affiduity in their dependents; and this remark will hold good, with *very few exceptions,*

ceptions, in almoft every inn from Yarmouth in Norfolk, to the land's end in Cornwall.

Under this eftablifhed truth, it is alfo an additional fact, that while the very refpectable clafs, whofe integrity I applaud, and whofe affiduity the public perceive and protect, are obtaining the very beft *corn* and *hay* that can be confumed upon the premifes, without refpect to the price of purchafe; not more from a defire to promote their hourly encreafing reputation, than to gratify the happy fenfation of inherent probity; the latter are conftantly procuring the hay and corn only, that can be purchafed at the VERY LOWEST PRICE, without a relative confideration to *quality, confcience*, or *reputation*.

Happy for the owners, much more happy for the fatigued and dejected horfes, if either poffeffed the good fortune or fagacity, to difcover the internal comforts by external appearance; nor can I conceive it would be bad policy in the very great numbers who conftantly travel, if they were to obtain by petition to parliament *a legal injunction*, that the SIGN *without* fhould be ftrictly emblematic

VOL. II.   A a   matic

matic of the treatment *within*; and thefe not correfponding, fhould be punifhed with the *lofs of licence* upon refpectable information. As it is, influenced by the power of external purity, we enter the gates of " AN ANGEL," and in a few minutes repentantly perceive we have been induced to encounter a DEVIL. Where we are taught to expect meeknefs from " THE LAMB," we frequently find the ferocity of A LION. At the " head of a KING," we meet accommodations for A COBLER. At a CASTLE, the manners of a COTTAGE. At the ROSE, we are furrounded with THORNS; and at the WHITE RAVEN, we difcover A ROOK.

Returning however from a flight digreffion to the fubject in agitation, I muft confefs, OSTLERS are a very ufeful body of men individually confidered; but long experience and attentive obfervation have rendered it an invariable rule with me, to adopt the good old maxim of " never trufting them *farther* than I can fee them;" and this upon the recollection of a *falfe manger* having been difcovered at a principal inn in the town of my nativity, in the days of juvenility; and the correfponding

ing declaration of a LEGERDEMAIN ADVEN-
TURER (at that time moſt applicably in
exhibition) whoſe ſalutary caution I have ever
retained: " LOOK SHARP, for if *your eyes*
are not quicker than *my hands* I ſhall certainly deceive you." This is a ſpecies of deception ſo conſtantly practiſed, and ſo happily enjoyed by the performers, that I make
it an invariable rule (by perſonal attendance)
to ſhield myſelf from the mortifying reflection of ſo much impoſition upon my pocket
or my underſtanding.

It ſhould be conſidered that ROAD HORSES
of every denomination are, from their conſtant work and great utility, entitled to a proportional degree of care and attention with
the moſt valuable horſes in the kingdom;
for though it is by no means neceſſary (but
evidently improper) they ſhould be in the
ſame high ſtate of condition as horſes appropriated to the higher ſpheres of racing and
hunting; yet there is a certain ſyſtematic uniformity in their mode of treatment, that regularly adhered to, will prove equally advantageous with one claſs, as the almoſt unbounded circumſpection ſo earneſtly recommended
with the other.

A a 2   For

For inſtance, very warm ſtables and a pro-
fuſion of body cloths are to be avoided, with
horſes that are neceſſarily deſtined to enter a
variety upon the road in conſtant travelling;
encountering the extremes of *heat* and *cold*,
the indifference of aliment, the various kinds
of water, and different modes of treatment.
Many of theſe, although not in the immediate need of ſuch large portions of NUTRI-
MENT as thoſe in the habit of more violent
exertions; yet they are entitled to all the uſeful minutiæ of ſtable diſcipline, that ſo clearly
contribute to the preſervation of health, in
horſes of a ſuperior deſcription.

Horſes coming under the denomination of
ROAD HORSES, or common hacks in occaſional excurſions and diurnal domeſtic employment, will ſupport themſelves in good
ſtate (with moderate gentle work) upon
three feeds of corn; on the contrary, horſes
of every kind, in conſtant work and exertions of magnitude, (as inceſſant journeying,
or travelling poſt) muſt be ſupplied, *at leaſt*,
with a peck of corn a day. Large and
ſtrong carriage horſes in perpetual work,
will

will require confiderably more, or become emaciated by lofs of flefh in frequent per-fpiration. Thefe rules are offered as a kind of general ftandard ; they muft, however, remain fubject to the conditional regulations of thofe who become individually interefted in the event.

There are numerous caufes to be affigned why horfes conftantly ufed in travelling (particularly in the winter) and fubject to all the viciffitudes of different ftabling upon the roads, moftly bear the appearance of invalids, and look fo very different from thofe kept under a fyftematic and invariable mode of management in private ftables. The degrees of deception, and various ills they have to encounter in many inns, are abfolutely incredible, to thofe unacquainted with *the arts* in fafhionable practice ; the deftructive negligence of *Oftlers,* the *badnefs of hay,* the *hardnefs* of *pump water,* and what is ftill more to be lamented, the SCARCITY OF CORN, render it a matter of aftonifhment how they are enabled to perform journies of fuch an amazing extent as they are perpetually deftined to.

A a 3

By

By way of prelude to the inftructions I conceive requifite, to form the mind of every young and inexperienced traveller; it cannot be confidered inapplicable to ftrengthen the inculcation by a fhort recital of an introductory fact that not long fince occurred in the neighbourhood of my prefent refidence : Where a farmer enjoyed his moiety of land at a very eafy rent, under an excellent landlord, and no immoderate oppreffion from parochial taxes ; and though he was univerfally known to be an honeft induftrious man, yet *repeated harvefts* produced nothing but additional deficiences ; in fhort, circumftances became annually more and more contracted, till DIRE NECESSITY compelled him to relinquifh both land and habitation, without having it in his power to accufe Providence of SEVERITY, or himfelf of NEGLECT.

He was foon fucceeded, at an advanced rent, by a man who was equally honeft, fober, and induftrious with himfelf ; who continued plodding on under the happy confolation of finding every harveft produce additional gain and accumulation of profit.

As

As FAME is seldom erroneous *in this particular*, his predecessor hearing of his success, under a considerable advance of rent, took the liberty of calling upon him, with a blunt but honest apology " for asking so impertinent a question; but it was, to be informed how he, who had the farm at a much easier rent, could not even pay that rent and subsist his family with all his care and œconomy; while his successor was not only evidently doing this, but daily increasing his stock from the superflux?" When the other replied, that the whole art of his success and improvement of the premises, consisted in nothing more than an invariable adherence to *two words* and their consequence; that when his predecessor held the farm, a too implicit confidence in and reliance upon his servants led him into unexpected and INVISIBLE losses. You, says he, always *ordered* your dependents to " Go" and do *this, that,* or the *other*; my plan is the very same as yours in every other respect but this; from the first hour of my coming into the farm it has been my constant maxim to say, " LET'S GO;" the *effect* of which has evidently occasioned the very

wide

wide difference between *your* circumftances and *mine*.

There certainly can be no doubt but the farmer's excellent maxim fhould be adopted by all thofe who rely too much upon the affected diligence of *oftlers*, and pretended fidelity of *fervants*; without a fingle confiftent reflection upon the caufe of their approaching every day nearer to poverty. For my own part, I am not at all afhamed to acknowledge, if my horfes are in higher condition as to external appearance, ftronger in the CHACE, or more refpectable upon the ROAD. than my neighbours, it is only to be attributed to the admirable admonition of " LET'S GO," under which incredible advantage of *perfonal fuper-intendance* I become fecurity for the certain execution of MY OWN ORDERS.

This to the inattentive or inconfiderate, may favor too ftrong of rigidity, and feem ftriking too much at the characters of fervants in general; however, the more prudent and difcriminating will know in what degree to admit the exception, concluding there may be fome entitled to a proper

proper extenfion of confidence; though taken in the aggregate, the proportion is fo exceedingly inferior, that *well-bought* EX-PERIENCE amply juftifies me in the opinion, that the greater number of dependents there are retained in any one family, (however fmall the fcale, or extenfive the eftablifhment,) the more the employer becomes the hourly prey of plunder and impofition.

Habituated to a belief of this fact, which it is beyond the power of either argument or fophiftry to difprove; I have long held in retention two excellent maxims (originally from high authority) that conftitute a ufeful TRIO, in conjunction with the emphatical PRECEPT of the farmer. That of "never putting off till *to-morrow* what can be done *to-day*;" or, "letting *another* do for you, what you can do for *yourfelf.*" Thefe rules conditionally adhered to, as much as circumftances, fituation, and relative confiderations will admit; would, I believe, have faved from ruin, THOUSANDS who have been depredated by the villainy of fervants, and now lament,

lament, in the moſt diſtreſſing indigence, their former inadvertency.

Theſe admonitions are introduced merely as a mirror worthy the accurate inſpection and remembrance of thoſe inconſiſtent beings, who, diſmounting at the different inns upon a journey, give their conſequential inſtructions to an oſtler, or perhaps a *ſtable boy*, and never condeſcend even to *look* upon the poor animal again, till neceſſarily produced for the continuance of his journey, at the end of twelve, twentyfour, or eight and forty hours. This almoſt incredible inſenſibility and ſelf-importance, brings to memory the pompoſity of a medical ſtudent freſh from the trammels of hoſpital attendance, and lectures upon OSTEOLOGY; whoſe head was ſo replete with anatomical phraſeology, that his mouth was never permitted to open but in a diſplay of profeſſional ability. For riding into one of the principal inns, in the firſt town in the county, and alighting from a poney of ſmall dimenſions, he vociferouſly reiterated the appellation of " OSTLER !" " SIR !" " diveſt my horſe of his *integuments !*"

Of the felf-fame dignity was poor WIGNELL, an inferior actor, but " *ftock King*," of Covent Garden Theatre for many years; whofe ftage confequence became fo habitual to him, he could never be divefted of it in the moft trifling occurrences of common life. At the conclufion of the winter feafon, when making his itinerant excurfion to join a company in the country for the fummer, he difmounted at an inn upon the road, and *ordering* proper proportions of corn and water for the BUCEPHALUS on which he rode, enjoyed himfelf moft luxurioufly upon the beft to be produced. When fatiate with good living, he depofited his pecuniary compenfation, and fallying forth, exclaimed moft theatrically for the " OSTLER ;" who appearing, the gueft approached him with his whip clenched in his hand (in the manner of a truncheon, like the Ghoft in Hamlet), ftill continuing to call upon the " OSTLER." The oftler recovering from the firft furprife, ventured, after fome trifling hefitation, to anfwer, but with *doubt* and *difmay*, " SIR !" " When my *fteed* has put a *period* to his *provender*, produce him."

This

This was a thunder ftroke to a man little read in *fcripture*, and a ftranger to *heroics*, particularly when accompanied with tragic EMPHASIS and ELOCUTION. John not knowing, and not being able to divine the meaning of this majeftic injunction, fcratched his head, and tremblingly re-echoed,. " SI, SI, R !" " When my *fteed* has put a *period* to his *provender*, produce him." " Upon my foul, Sir, I don't know what you mean !" " Why, you fcoundrel ! when my horfe has *eat his corn*, bring him out of the ftable." Whether he had really been put in poffeffion of *any corn at all*, was a matter of no PERSONAL CONCERN to poor WIGNELL, provided he had the immaculate affurance of the *Oftler*, that it was all confumed ; and this, it is much to be regretted, is the invariable cuftom of numbers, who deftitute of the finer feelings, and perfect ftrangers to the enlivening rays of HUMANITY, are open to no other fenfation, than the predominant gratification of felf-prefervation.

Returning, however, to the management of ROAD HORSES, whether on a journey

of

of continuance, or in their daily work at home, and refident in their own ftables, the fame care and attention are equally neceffary; I have ever (feelingly) found, SERVANTS at home require the fame circumfpection and fuperintendance as OSTLERS abroad; and happy that man, if *one there is*, who through life has had well-founded reafon to be of a different opinion; if fo, he is entitled to my beft congratulations, for poffeffing fo valuable a novelty.

Horfes of this defcription have every claim with others to the fame regularity of ftable difcipline; they fhould be at all times as equally prepared for a journey, as their fuperiors for the chace; the faddle has as great a right to be complete and fit eafy, and the fhoes to be as firm as the firft hunter in the kingdom. They are at all times entitled to fubftantial dreffing, good foft water, and proper exercife; their legs and heels to be well wafhed from dirt, and rubbed dry, in the winter feafon; their feet to be picked, ftopped, and hoofs oiled, at all feafons of the year;

and

and their hay and corn as methodically given, and as good in its kind (if poffible to be obtained, which in moft inns it is not) as to thofe of fuperior qualifications. And thefe peculiar attentions become the more neceffary, if the owner, from that innate monition that is an ornament to human nature; or the prevalence of fafhion in external appearance, wifhes him to move with pleafure to himfelf, and credit to his mafter.

There are various matters of general concern, that require a little animadverfion: Firft, the indifcreet act of riding a horfe to the end of his journey in a ftate of violent perfpiration, to be then led about in the hands of an Oftler, till *he cools*; and this at all times of the year, without the leaft refpect to feafons. The abfurdity is fo palpable, under the defined effect of obftructed perfpiration fo repeatedly introduced, that an additional line is not required upon the fubject: but that the inconfiftency of fuch practice may more forcibly affect thofe who perfevere only from inadvertency, and others who are

are fufficiently humble to imbibe inftruction ; let it be perfectly underftood, that
any man riding very faft, without a fubftantial reafon, is never by the *impartial
fpectator* taken for a KING or a *Conjurer.*

But left my unfupported opinion fhould
have no weight with fuch HIGHFLYING
gentry, I beg to advance a fenfible remark
of a neighbouring friend (very recently
made) who, in ferious converfation, affured me, " he never faw a man *gallop*
into or out of a town, but he was clearly
convinced, the horfe was not HIS OWN, or
the rider was either *a fool* or *a madman.*"
To this very fair and candid inference, I
am induced to add another corroboration
of public opinion, upon what they conceive the moft ftriking proof of their courage and refpectability. An old farmer
within three miles of my own refidence,
having difmiffed a brother of the faculty
who formerly attended his family, gave me
this very concife reafon for fo doing ; " I
did not choofe he fhould attend my family any longer, for he always rides fo
faft, I am fure HE NEVER THINKS." Is it
poffible,

poffible, can it be hardly credible, that any rational compofition, after giving thefe truths (that have fallen from old and experienced obfervers) a moment's reflection, will ever lay himfelf open to the feverity of farcafms, or rather juft contemptuous reproofs, that inftantly conftitute him a fool or a madman in the eyes of all the world? Under confiderations of fo much weight, I can have but little doubt that every *random traveller*, (not totally callous to the dictates of prudence and difcretion) to whofe rumination thefe hints may become fubfervient; will, in future, diveft himfelf of his ÆROSTATIC FUROR, and conclude his ftage or journey by fuch gradual declination of fpeed for the laft two or three miles, as may bring his horfe *tolerably cool* into the proper receptacle, without perfevering in a public proof of folly, always productive of danger and certain contempt.

As it is fo evidently proper to ride a horfe very moderately at the conclufion of a journey, fo it muft prove equally neceffary at the beginning. When a horfe is brought

out

out of the ftable with the ftomach and inteftines expanded with food and excrement,
he cannot encounter RAPID EXERTION without much difficulty and temporary inconvenience, till the inteftinal accumulation is confiderably reduced and carried off by repeated
evacuations; the work of digeftion fhould
alfo be gradually effected to relieve the ftomach, and take from the preffure that muft
inevitably fall upon the lobes of the lungs,
(reftraining their natural elafticity) under
which the horfe muft move with a load of
difquietude till fuch weight is progreffively
removed.

The certainty of this fact every reader of
no more than common fagacity will difcover,
without further information from me; when
I refer him to his recollection, for the great
difficulty a horfe encounters, when put into
HASTY ACTION, after receiving his portion of *food* and *water*, either at morning,
noon, or night. From this remark directly
branches another, equally worthy the confideration of travellers; that is, the almoft
univerfal abfurdity of giving, or *rather ordering* their horfes a pail of cold water (ufually

in inn yards from the pump) in the morning, sometimes before, (which is ridiculous in the extreme) but generally *immediately after* they have swallowed their corn ; upon an erroneous supposition, that upon such ACCUMULATED STUFFING, they will be enabled to surmount all the difficulties of a long and fatiguing journey.

Upon the inconsistency of this practice, I beg to appeal only to the unprejudiced remembrance of those who have unthinkingly adopted it; whether horses thus loaded, do not travel for some miles with the greatest seeming labour and inconvenience? Admitting this position without a single exception, there cannot be a remaining doubt, but those horses, commencing their journey almost immediately after the stomach becomes expanded with the accustomed portion of hay and corn; had with much more propriety proceed a few miles gently on the road, and take their water at a soft STANDING POND, or POOL, when the frame (by preceding evacuations) is more adapted to receive it. But even in this alternative, proper discrimination is absolutely necessary; for horses, either on a journey or

in

in common exercife, fhould never be permitted to drink at all in *fharp fhallow ftreams,* that run over a rufty gravel, or through a black peaty foil; they are equally harfh, and feldom or never fail to have a fevere effect upon the inteftinal canal, in producing *fret* or *cholic* in a greater or lefs degree, and fetting the coat by a fudden collapfion of the cutaneous pores in a few minutes after ufe.

To enumerate the minutiæ of MANAGEMENT, and bring it into a concife and fingle point of view, I heartily (and upon experimental proof of the advantage) recommend every perfon upon a journey, *whether long or fhort,* who takes up his temporary refidence AT INNS, to make it his invariable rule TO SEE (by either himfelf or fervant) that his horfes are *dreffed, fed,* and *watered;* their heels wafhed, feet ftopped, hoofs oiled, and his equipments or apparatus, whether for riding or driving, examined *as to their fafety,* every night or morning, if not at every ftage; perhaps the latter may always prove the moft eligible, for thofe who will compound at a very trifing degree of additional trouble,

B b 2

to

to avoid the poffibility of unexpected danger or difappointment.

To infure the execution of all which, with the lefs reluctance on the part of your dependents, let it be ever predominant in the mind, " to do as you would be done unto ;" LIBERALITY judicioufly exerted is the beft fecurity for a cheerful execution of your wifhes. It fhould be forcibly impreffed upon the mind of every traveller, who wifhes to become a gueft of refpectability, that " the labourer is worthy of his hire," and the hope of reward fweetens labour. Upon the OSTLER, the WAITER, and the CHAMBERMAID, depends not only your comfort but your fafety; and it is fo completely in the *junction of the trio*, to render your armed chair eafy, or replete with the thorns of difquietude, that it will be not only neceffary you treat them with becoming civility, divefted of the difgufting pride of perfonal oftentation ; but take care to beftow fuch *expreffive marks* of your approbation, as will fufficiently influence them to confider you upon every future occafion, more the domeftic friend than the cafual ftranger.

In

3

In pecuniary compenfations of this kind it is ridiculous to be on the penurious fide of gratification ; a fingle fhilling very frequently, IN THEIR OPINIONS, conftitutes the line of diftinction between " A GENTLEMAN" and " A BLACKGUARD ;" then who would encounter

> " The infolence of office, and the fpurns
> " That patient merit of th' unworthy takes,"

when " a good name," with a profufion of adulation, may be purchafed for fo paltry a confideration. In fhort, although the expences attendant upon the conveniences of fuch receptacles conftitute a tax of enormity ; yet if you wifh to infure your own comfort, with the fafety of your horfe, you have no alternative but to confider them debts of honour that muft be paid.

Before we bid adieu to the fubject of road horfes, it cannot prove inapplicable to introduce a few remarks upon the inconfiftency of wafhing the bodies of poft and ftage horfes all over with *cold water*, fo foon as they are taken out of their harnefs, when in the higheft ftate of perfpiration. This cuftom is become

B b 3

come fo univerfal, that we perceive its adoption
in almoft every inn yard of eminence through
the kingdom : That I may, however, avoid
the accufation of rafhly condemning a practice
fo numeroufly fupported, I fhall only ftart
fuch matters of opinion for due deliberation,
as may more materially concern thofe interefted in the confequence.

That is, whether it is poffible to believe,
(after a moment's reflection) that a horfe who
has gone ten, fifteen, or twenty miles with
great exertion, and is brought in with the perfpirable matter paffing off in ftreams; can be
completely plunged into a torrent of COLD
WATER, without at leaft the *very great pro-*
bability of deftructive confequences, from inftantaneoufly clofing the cuticular pores, and
inevitably locking up the whole mafs of fe-
creted perfpirative matter in a ftate of temporary ftagnation ?

In this unnatural fhock the conftitution
becomes the criterion of decifion, the whole
afpect depending entirely upon the ftate of the
blood; if the horfe fhould be luckily free from
every trait of difeafe, and rather *below* than
above

above himfelf in condition, difplaying a ftate of purity in appearance, nature may, under fuch favourable circumftances, prove herfelf adequate to the tafk of abforption, and it may be again received into the circulation, no ill confequences becoming perceptible : But fhould the veffels have been before overload-ed, and the blood in a ftate of VISCIDITY, very great danger muft inevitably enfue ; for the perfpirative matter thus preternaturally thrown upon the circulation, after acquiring by its ftagnation a proportional tenacity, muft render the whole fyftem liable to fudden in-flammation upon increafing the blood's mo-tion to the leaft degree of velocity.

To the perfuafive force of thefe probable effects, I have long fince become the greater convert, by attentively adverting to the great number of THOSE HORSES that fo fuddenly drop dead upon the road, in the very next ftage after having undergone fuch unnatural ablution. To the rational or fcientific ob-ferver, the caufe of thefe deaths does not require a momentary inveftigation ; the fyftem of CIRCULATION, DERIVATION, REPLE-TION, and REVULSION are too well under-

B b 4   ftood

ftood to hefitate a moment in pronouncing fuch fudden deaths to be generally occafioned by the means already affigned : The phyfical procefs of which repulfion of perfpirative matter, and its effects upon various habits, are too minutely explained under the heads of different difeafes, in many parts of our former volume, to render farther difquifition in the leaft neceffary.

For my own part, ever open to intellectual improvement and conftantly courting con- viction, I moft anxioufly wifh to be informed, through the channel of fyftematic impartia- lity, what can be *hoped*, *wifhed*, or *expected* from a proceeding fo entirely new ; that can- not be more confiftently obtained by the ut- moft extent of friction properly perfevered in, with the ufual modes of WISPING, BRUSH- ING, and CLEANING, as in general ufe in almoft every ftable of uniformity in the king- dom. Nor can I at all conceive, as every thing that can be required relative to condi- tion, labour, and appearance is to be effected by means divefted of danger ; why fuch un- juftifiable modes need be brought into prac- tice, without a fingle confiftent idea to juftify

their

their introduction for either improvement or utility.

Having formerly made some few observations upon the convenience of Public Repositories for the sale of horses by auction; I am induced, from a recent discovery, to add a single remark upon one of their *local laws*, indicative of great apparent probity in the proprietors of such receptacles, but replete with danger to those, who consign valuable horses for sale, should the rules so made be persevered in. Since the publication of my former volume, a friend (upon my making an occasional journey to London) begged me to execute the commission of selling a sound five year old mare at one of the most fashionable repositories in the metropolis. Reaching London the day preceding the sale, and giving my instructions, I returned in the morning, and after amusing myself upon different parts of the premises, accidently approached the PULPIT; upon which was affixed literary information, " that persons selling horses WARRANTED SOUND on *a Monday* were entitled to the money *on Friday*, and those so sold and warranted on *a Thursday* might receive payment

payment on the following *Monday*; if in the mean time fuch horfe or horfes were not returned AS UNSOUND." The palpable abfurdity of propofitions fo ridiculous and unjuft inftantly deranged all my premeditated plan of proceeding; for upon re-confidering my commiffion and the conditions of fale, I found if the mare was fold at the hammer I had not only to make *a waiting job* of four days in London for payment, but the chance of A LAME MARE at the expiration of that time, inftead of the money. For the purchafer poffeffing the privilege of riding her for fo long, might fo do to any diftance, or any degree of diftrefs; and not approving her in *every action,* had only to confer the favour of *a blow* upon any particular part, to occafion temporary pain and limping, that might juftify a return under the plea of *unfoundnefs,* rendering the feller a dupe to the force of credulity and REPOSITORICAL INTEGRITY.

Under the weight of indignation, that naturally arofe from ferious reflection, upon fuch an evident want of confiftency in mutual conditions that we are naturally to conclude, SHOULD fix the ftandard of EQUITY, and

and prevent unfair preponderation in favour of *either buyer or seller* ; I returned the mare to the owner without exposing her to sale, with an invariable determination, never to sell a horse of even TEN POUNDS value, where the purchaser may not only possess the privilege, but *sufficient time* to render him a complete cripple, by hard riding or bad management, leaving me no consolation but my own acquiescence and extreme folly for repentance.

Taking into consideration the very tedious and expensive litigations that have been carried on in our courts of law, upon the subject of horses proving *unsound* some time after sale and delivery ; I think it necessary (after proper reference to the definition of the word " SOUND," in the early part of the former volume,) to introduce my own method of disposal, where I conceive the horse to be perfectly healthy and entirely sound at the moment of delivery.

A learned Peer upon one bench, may, under sanction of an eminent situation, and the advantage of coining *a new law* to answer anfwer every particular purpofe, dictatorially infinuate to a jury, " that a horfe fhould continue found for a certain number of *days, weeks*, or *months* after the purchafe ;" and fix upon a ftipulated fum for what he has condefcended to term " A SOUND PRICE ;" afcertaining fuch opinion an invariable criterion for all future decifions in Weftminfter-Hall : Or a worthy Baron upon another, " that a man may *lawfully* correct his wife with a ftick no bigger than his THUMB." But however accurate fuch calculations may have been made by the very high and refpectable authorities I allude to, they cannot be more free from cafual *exceptions*, than the great infinity of rules where EXCEPTIONS are always admitted.

However, as I confefs myfelf one of thofe never implicitly bound merely by *matter of opinion*, with an utter averfion to difpofing of horfes in Weftminfter-Hall, and experimentally convinced how very fuddenly horfes *fall lame* without a vifible caufe ; as well as how frequently they are attacked with acute difeafe and *rapidly carried off* without any particular reafon to be collected EVEN FROM DISSEC

TION ;

TION : Under the influence of thefe predominant facts, I have long fince adopted a certain invariable mode of difpofal, that I confcientioufly recommend, to prevent difgrace
on one fide, or diffatisfaction on the other.

My method is equally concife and decifive : If the horfe is unequivocally SOUND,
I am perfectly content to warrant him fo,
even upon oath if required, to the hour of
DELIVERY, but not a *fingle hour* beyond it ;
for let it be held in memory, he is as liable
to become *lame, difeafed*, or a fubject of
diffolution, in that very hour, as in any
other of his life.——I am equally willing to
fhow all his paces with hounds, or on the
road, (according to his appropriation) but
not mounted by *a ftranger*, of whofe qualifications *in riding* I know as little as he
does of my horfe in *temper* and *action* ; and
confequently, from a want of congeniality
between the natural difpofition of *one*, and
correfponding pliability of the *other*, the
horfe might be fhown to palpable difadvantage. For it may be relied on, and accepted as a certain fact, that almoft every
horfe will move in another ftile, and difplay
a very

a very different figure, when croffed by one that he is accuftomed to, who knows his tendencies, and the ftate of his mouth, than under the hands of one to whom he is totally unknown; all which they have natural fagacity to difcover, in a much greater degree than generally believed by thofe who have had but flender opportunities of attending to their perfections.

The   T U R F,

That has totally diffipated fome of the moft fplendid fortunes in a very few years, and left the poffeffors to lament in INDIGENCE, the fatal effects of their credulity, and the folly of infection; is entitled to fuch few remarks as appertain to the prevalence of a fafhion that has, within a very fhort fpace of years, involved not only numbers of the moft EMINENT CHARACTERS, but *hundreds of inferior,* in the general ruin. For the laft half century this rage has been fo very predominant that great numbers even

of

of the commercial world could not with-
ftand the force of temptation; to have a
horfe or two IN TRAINING has been an
object of the higheft ambition, to the gratification of which, every other profpect or
purfuit has been rendered fubfervient. The
contagion has been in its effects fo delufive,
that Lottery Office Keepers and Pawnbrokers
have been racing againft the horfes of Peers
of the realm, to the inevitable accumulation
of DEBTS, the defrauding of CREDITORS,
and the promoting of BANKRUPTCIES.
This is not calculated to create furprife,
when it is not only recollected in rumination,
but confirmed by time and experience, that
nothing but a fortune of immenfity can ftand
againft the enormous expence of BREEDING
and TRAINING; the fluctuating uncertainty
of the produce; and laftly, what is ftill more
to be dreaded, the *innate villainy* and *ftudied
deception* of the fubordinate claffes, with
whom your HONOUR and PROPERTY are
eventually entrufted; and upon whofe *caprice,
intereft, villainy, or integrity,* you muft unavoidably depend, to carry your purpofes into
execution.

9

However

However ftrange and unpromifing this delineation may appear to the young and
inexperienced fportfman, (who having no
guile in his own difpofition, does not fufpect it in others) yet the projected villainies
are fo numerous, and refined to fo many
different degrees of deception, that in the
prefent ftate of *fporting purification,* it is almoft impoffible for any man to train and
run a horfe, or make a fingle bet upon their
fuccefs, without falling into one of the innumerable plots that will be laid for his deftruction. Exclufive of the experimental
proofs we fhall have occafion to introduce
in corroboration of this remark, it may not
be out of point to obferve, that a late noble
Lord, within my own memory, was fo well
convinced of this fact, that when in the abfolute poffeffion of a STABLE OF WINNERS,
he totally relinquifhed a purfuit of fo much
pleafure, and fold off his ftud, rather than
continue the ftanding prey of premeditated
plunder ; convinced by long and attentive
experience, no moderate fortune or common
fagacity could fhield him from the joint
rapacity of dependents, who were to parti-
cipate

cipate in the conftant depredation upon an individual.

To this prudent decifion, he was juftly influenced by the eagerly expected return of his training groom from a fummer expedition, with three running horfes of fome eminence, that had in their excurfion of little more than four months, obtained poffeffion of feven fifty pound plates. But after having received the different prizes, and difcharged all contingent expences, this FAITHFUL STEWARD, by the dint of arithmetical proficiency, brought his Mafter in debtor, *upon the balance*, upwards of fifty pounds. This impofition (or rather robbery) too palpable not to be difcovered, his Lordfhip, with a degree of liberality fuperior to perfonal altercation, immediately obliterated, and then declared his inflexible determination to difcontinue both BREEDING and TRAINING, a refolution he fteadily perfevered in to the end of his life; nor has it been renewed by either of his fucceffors, though there are in the family manfion, as excitements, feveral capital paintings of many of the firft horfes of their time, that had been bred by their different predeceffors.

This judicious refignation proved only a voluntary prelude to the wonderful anni-hilation of property that has compulfively followed with thofe of lefs prudence, pe-netration, or refolution ; in corroboration of which, we are prevented by delicacy alone, from an enumeration of even the initials only of the names of many eminent and ennobled charafters, (formerly poffeffed of princely fortunes) who now *fubfift merely* upon the fcanty favings from the wreck of indifcretion : ftripped of the numerous ftud and pompous appendages, to which their titles were blazoned forth in various lifts, of " The famous high-bred running cattle," as well as the annual " Racing Calendar." Some few of the Right Ho-nourable Adventurers have efcaped the " general ruin," and fortunately retain their poffeffions and undiminifhed ftuds ; but they are fo conftantly contracting in num-ber, that they ferve only to eftablifh the admitted exception to rules, in which we

may

may fairly infer their immenfe propertics to have operated as preventatives.

This fport, that has for many years been fo exceedingly prevalent, is at length declining very faft among the middle and inferior claffes of people; and of this diminution the annual contribution of two guineas each to government is a fufficient proof, when it is known, that all the horfes that RUN, PAID, or RECEIVED FORFEIT, in the united kingdoms laft year, did not exceed eight hundred: a number that does not much furpafs the averaged half of horfes fupported in training fome few years paft; a circumftance that requires little farther corroboration, than the numerous plates advertifed in different parts, for the two or three laft years, that were never run for, " *for want of horfes.*"

This falling off may be juftly attributed to a combination of obftacles; the conftantly encreafing expence of TRAINING, the minifterial TAX, the profeffional duplicity (or rather * *family deception*) of RI-

* Gamblers are known by the appellation of " The Black Legged Family."

DERS,

DERS, the heavy expenditure unavoidably attendant upon travelling from one feat of fport to another; the very great probability of *accidents* or *breaking down* in running, with a long train of uncertainties, added to the infamous practices of the " Black Legged" fraternity, in perpetual intercourfe and affociation with both TRAINERS and RIDERS; leaving the cafual fportfman a very flender chance of winning *one* bet in *ten*, where any of this *worthy fociety* are concerned; which they generally are by fome means, through the medium of occafional emiffaries, mercenary agents, or ftable dependants, in conftant pay for the proftitution of every truft that has been implicitly repofed in them by their too credulous employers.

Such incontrovertible truths may perhaps appear matters of mere conjecture and fpeculation to the young and inexperienced, who will undoubtedly believe with reluctance, what is fo evidently calculated to difcourage the predominance of inclination; and not having explored the regions of difcovery, they may be induced to flatter themfelves with an opinion, that fuch reprefentation is a delufion
intended

intended much more to entertain than communicate inftruction. However, that the bufinefs may be elucidated in fuch way, as will prove moft applicable to the nature of the cafe and the patience of the reader; it will be neceffaay to afford their practices fuch explanation, as may render the facility of execution more familiar to the imagination of thofe, whofe fituations in life, or contracted opportunities, may have prevented their being at all informed upon the fubject in agitation.

That thefe acts of villainy may be the better underftood, it becomes applicable to obferve, that it is the perfevering practice of THE FAMILY, to have four, five, or fix known good runners in their poffeffion; though for the convenience and greater certainty of public depredation, they pafs as the diftinct property of different members: but this is by no means the cafe, for they are as much the joint ftock of *the party*, as is the ftock in trade of the firft firm in the city. The fpeed and bottom of thefe horfes are as accurately known to each individual of the brotherhood, and they are in general (without an unexpected accident which fometimes happens) as well convinced *before starting*, whether they can beat their competitors, as if the race was abfolutely determined.

This, however, is only the neceffary groundwork of deception, upon which every part of the fuperftructure is to be raifed : as they experimentally know how little money is to be got by *winning*, they feldom permit that to become an object of momentary confideration ; and being no flaves to the fpecious delufions of HONOUR, generally make their market by the *reverfe*, but more particularly where they are the leaft expected *to lofe :* that is, they fucceed beft in their general depredations by *lofing* where their horfes are the favourites at high odds after a heat or two, when expected to *win to a certainty*, which they as PRUDENTLY take care to prevent.

This bufinefs, to infure fuccefs and emolument, is carried on by fuch a combination of villainy ; fuch a fympathetic chain of horrid machination, as it is much to be lamented could ever enter the minds of degenerate men for the purpofes of deftruction.

3 The

The various modes of practice and impofition are too numerous and extenfive to admit of general explanation; the purport of the prefent *epitome* or contracted defcription being intended to operate merely as a guard to thofe, who are totally unacquainted with the *infamy* of the party, whofe MERITS we mean to defcribe.

The principal (that is, the oftenfible proprietor of the horfe for the day) is to be found in the centre of the " BETTING RING," previous to the ftarting of the horfe, furrounded by the fporting multitude; amongft whom his emiffaries place themfelves to perform their deftined parts in the acts of villainy regularly carried on upon thefe occafions; but more particularly at all the meetings within thirty or forty miles of the metropolis. In this confpicuous fituation, he forms a variety of PRETENDED BETS with his confederates, in favour of his own horfe; fuch bait the unthinking byftanders immediately fwallow, and proceeding upon this fhew of confidence, *back him themfelves:* thefe offers are immediately accepted to any amount by the emiffaries before-mentioned,

and

and is in fact no more than a palpable robbery; as the horfe, it is already determined
BY THE FAMILY, is *not to win*, and the
money *fo betted* is as certainly their own as
if already decided.

This part of the bufinefs being tranfact-
ed, a new fcene of tergiverfation becomes
neceffary; the horfe being mounted, the
rider is whifpered by the *nominal owner* to
win the firft heat if he can; this it is frequently in his power *to do eafy*, when he is
confequently backed at ftill *increafed odds* as
the expected winner; all which propofed
bets are inftantly taken by the emiffaries, or
rather principals *in the firm*: when, to
fhew us the verfatility of FORTUNE, and the
viciffitudes of the turf, he very *unexpectedly*
becomes A LOSER, or perhaps *runs out of the
courfe*, to the feigned difappointment and
affected forrow of the owner; who publicly
declares he has loft fo many " fcore pounds
upon the race," whilft his confederates are
individually engaged in collecting *their cer-
tainties*, previous to the CASTING UP
STOCK, at the general rendezvous in the
evening.

To

To this plan there is a direct alternative, if there fhould be no chance (from his being fufficiently a favourite) of laying on money in this way; they then take the longeft odds they can obtain that he wins, and regulate or vary their betting by the event of each heat, winning if they can, or *lofing to a certainty,* as beft fuits the bets they have laid; which is accurately known by a pecuniary confultation between the heats. From another degree of undifcoverable duplicity their greater emoluments arife: For inftance, letting a horfe of capital qualifications WIN and LOSE almoft alternately at different places, as may be moft applicable to the betting for the day; dependent entirely upon the ftate of public opinion, but to be ultimately decided by the latent villainy of the parties more immediately concerned.

Thefe, like other matters of magnitude, are not to be rendered infallible, without the neceffary agents; that, like the fmaller wheels of a curious piece of mechanifm, contribute their portion of power to give action to the whole. So true is the ancient adage, " birds of a feather flock together,"

that

that RIDERS may be selected, who will prove inviolably faithful to the dictates of this party; that *could not* or *would not* reconcile an honourable attachment to the first noblemen in the kingdom. These are the infernal deceptions and acts of villany upon THE TURF, that have driven noblemen, gentlemen, and sportsmen of honour, from what are called *country courfers* to their asylum of NEWMARKET; where, by the exclusion of THE FAMILY from their clubs, and their horses from their SUBSCRIPTIONS, SWEEPSTAKES and MATCHES, they render themselves invulnerable to the *often envenomed* shafts of the most premeditated (and in general well executed) villainy.

Without entering into a tedious description of the many possible means by which depredations are committed upon the property of individuals, whom fashion or inclination prompts to sport their money upon such occasions; yet to render these villainous practices more familiar to the minds of those who may incredulously doubt the possibility of deceptions of this kind, instances must be adduced to establish the certainty,

of

of which there has been too many public proofs, to require the fpecification of any particular fact for the purpofe. It may fuffice to obferve, it is univerfally known fuch villainies have been repeatedly difcovered; where the owners have been notorioufly difqualified by advertifements, from ever running their horfes, and thofe riders from riding, at the places where they have been fo juftly ftigmatized, and fo properly held in the utmoft contempt.

Upon fo precarious a tenure does every fporting man of fpirit retain his hope of fuccefs, that I will be bound to verify the affertion by innumerable inftances; that no man living can BREED, TRAIN, and RUN his horfes to infure even a probability of emolument, by any honourable means whatever. Noblemen and Gentlemen of immenfe fortunes, to whom it' is an amufement, and who never know the want of annual receipts, in a repetition of thoufands; may indulge themfelves in a gratification of their predominant wifhes, and feel no ill effect from a variety of loffes, or perpetual expenditure.

It

It is not fo with thofe of inferior property
and fituation ; as may be plainly perceived
in the great number who become rotationally infected with the experiment of training for *one fummer*, but never *repeat it*.
This is not at all to be wondered at, when
we recollect, that after all the expence,
trouble, and anxiety, you have expofed
yourfelf to, for the *very diftant* chance of
obtaining a fifty pound plate or two, with
various deductions ; you are at laft under
the unavoidable neceffity of refigning the
bridle into the hands of a man, who may
perhaps prove one of *the greateft rafcals*
among the groupe we have already defcribed.
For when thus felected for fo important a
truft, it may fo happen, *you* have never feen
him before ; nor may *he* ever fee *you* again:
On the contrary, he may be connected with
a little hoft of colleagues upon the courfe,
with whom he is perpetually concerned in
acts of reciprocal kindnefs and joint depredation.

From fuch dangerous delegation, you can
form (upon reflection) no hope of fuccefs ;
unlefs your horfe, by the rider's *endeavour*

to

to win, fhould ·prove productive of bets,
beft fuiting the convenience of the FA-
MILY. However, to render this perfectly
clear, let us confirm the fact by a ftate-
ment not to be mifunderftood. Suppofe,
the owner of a horfe compenfates a rider,
that he engages from an idea of his fuperior ability, reputed integrity, or upon
recommendation, with a promife of five
guineas certain to ride according to inftructions *for each heat,* and a conditional *five*
or *ten* extra, if he wins. What can be the
utmoft emolument to him by winning?
Why, as before ftated, either TEN or FIF-
TEEN guineas! While, on the contrary,
if the horfe is of character and qualifications, and the odds run a little in his
favour for the laft heat; the induftrious
efforts of the rider's confederates, who are
taking thofe very odds *laid upon the horfe,*
(that it is already pre-determined fhall lofe)
they accumulate and divide much larger fums
to a certainty, without the chance of lofing
a fingle guinea.

I fhall not defcend to an enumeration of
a variety of practices that render plunder
equally

equally fafe from detection; as giving a horfe water in the night previous to the day of running; or throwing *a mild ca-tbartic,* or *ftrong diuretic* into the body, to produce indifpofition, and prevent the POSSIBILITY of a horfe WINNING, when it is determined by the CABINET COUN-SEL, that it is for the *general good* he muft LOSE. If any rational being, any generous unfufpecting fportfman, or any juvenile no-viciate, has the moft flender doubt re-maining of thefe practices, let me render the matter decifive, and bring it to a ne-ceffary conclufion, by a fingle queftion that will not require a moment's difcuffion in reply.

By what other means than thofe al-ready defcribed between the FAMILY and THE RIDERS, have the numbers that are well known, and that we conftantly fee in the *height of bufinefs* in every popu-lous betting ring, arifen to a ftate of opu-lence? What can have exalted men who were bankrupts in trade; poft-chaife drivers, hair dreffers, waiters, footmen, nay, the loweft clafs of gamblers, (that ab-

folutely

folutely raifed contributions among the moft wretched, by even the infamous practices of " *pricking in the belt,*" and " *huftling in the hat,*") to their PHAETONS, *horfes in training,* and confpicuous feats in the firft fafhionable BETTING STANDS, (among the moft eminent characters in the kingdom) but fuch acts of premeditated and deep laid villainy, as no man living can be guarded againft, if he embarks or ventures his property amongft *a fet of ruffians,* that are not only a notorious peft to fociety, but a dangerous nuifance and obftruction to one of the nobleft diverfions our kingdom has to boaft.

Under fuch numerous difadvantages, it muft prove palpably clear to every ob-ferver, that none but fportfmen with for-tunes of the firft magnitude, can confcien-tioufly enjoy the pleafure of BREEDING, TRAINING, and RUNNING their horfes, without the perpetual dread of approach-ing ruin; in fact, of this fuch a repetition of proofs have tranfpired within the laft twenty years, that the leaft defcriptive corroboration becomes totally unneceffary.

For

For my own part, I am decifively and experimentally convinced, no man in moderate circumftances, who cannot afford a daily proftitution of property for the inceffant gratification of dependent fharks on one hand, and the perpetual fupply of deceptive villains on the other, can never expect to become the winner of MATCH, PLATE, or SWEEPSTAKES, unlefs he happily poffeffes the means and fituation to go through the bufinefs of *training* under his own roof, and *riding his own horfe*; or fixing firm reliance upon fome faithful domeftic properly qualified, totally unconnected with the contaminating crew, whofe conduct we have fo accurately delineated, without an additional ray of exaggeration. But as my declaration of *proof* collected from EXPERIMENTAL CONVICTION, may not be generally accepted as fufficiently authentic, without fome more powerful evidence than bare fuperficial affertion; I muft beg permiffion to conclude thefe obfervations, upon the prefent ftate and various impofitions of THE TURF, with the communication of a few perfonal occurrences, that I doubt not will contribute

fome

fome weight to the opinions I have fubmitted to public confideration.

In the fummer of feventeen hundred feventy-five, I ran a match of four miles, carrying twelve ftone, (with a gelding got by BROOMSTICK) againft a mare, the property of a gentleman of confiderable fortune in the county of Effex, for fifty guineas. His extenfive property was confpicuous in an elegant manfion, a paddock of deer, a pack of harriers, and a liberal fubfcription to a neighbouring pack of fox hounds. That we might be equally free from even a chance of the deception in *riding* I have juft defcribed; we trufted to our own abilities in jockeyfhip, for a decifion in which *I conceived* our honour and property were EQUALLY concerned. The match, however, was decided againft him with *perfect eafe,* upon which he loft fome confiderable bets; but in the mortification of his difappointment, affecting to believe it was won with much difficulty, he propofed to run the fame match on that day fortnight, upon my confenting to give him five pounds, or, in other words, to reduce his weight to *eleven ſtone nine*. This was inſtantly acceded to, and many bets made in conſequence, among our neighbouring friends; but previous to the day of running, having accepted an invitation to his houſe, he there *moſt honourably* offered to pay me the five and twenty guineas, *before the race*, if " I would obligingly condeſcend to let him WIN." I have a firm and anxious hope, that every ſportſman of integrity, whoſe feelings vibrate in uniſon with my own, and who reads this propoſition with the indignation it is recited; will do me the juſtice to conſider it more proper, that he ſhould *conceive*, than becoming in me to *relate*, the particulars of my behaviour upon ſuch occaſion. It muſt ſuffice to ſay, I rode over the courſe without a companion; and as the match was made PLAY or PAY, received the payment for my conſolation. There are numerous and very powerful reaſons, why I forbear to make a ſingle remark upon this buſineſs; leaving it entirely, with its infinity of *annual ſimilitudes*, to the different impreſſions it may make upon the

PRIN-

PRINCIPLES of the different readers to whom it will become a fubject.

This was only a fingle attack, confequently parried with much greater eafe, than when affailed by an almoft incredible combination of villainy, in running a match for the fame fum four years fince, upon one of the moft populous and fafhionable courfes in the kingdom. But having *then*, as *before*, the fame invariable opinion of the duplicity practifed in TRAINING and RIDING, I had never permitted the mare out of my poffeffion, or from under my own infpection, from the hour fhe was matched to run; or intended her to be rode by any other perfon, than a lad of my own. that (literally fpeaking) I initiated in ftable management and *trained* with the mare for the purpofe.

Thus entrenched by prudence, and fortified by experience, it was impoffible for thofe concerned againft me, either by their numerous emiffaries, or induftrious adherents, to obtain the requifite intelligence of *trials*,

fweats,

fweats, or in fact any neceſſary information, by which their intentional villainy could be promoted with a probability of ſucceſs. But as adventurers of this complexion are never diſconcerted by trifling obſtacles, it will create no ſmall degree of ſurpriſe, to thoſe not at all appriſed of the various ſhifts, inventions, and ſchemes of villainy in conſtant practice upon the TURF; to be informed of the innumerable and remote contrivances, eternally adopted for the promotion of robbery and depredation upon others, as well as the execution of their intents upon me, which, however, very fortunately did not ſucceed.

On the day of running, having removed my mare from my own ſtable to a recluſe and convenient houſe within two miles of the courſe; locked her up by five in the morning, and conſigned my lad to his pillow, (to prevent either *converſation* or *communication,*) I was almoſt immediately enquired for by *a jockey* of ſome eminence, whoſe ability is held in tolerable eſtimation. Being juſt then in the act of taking breakfaſt, and the parlour door having been

left

left a very little open, I could juſt diſtinguiſh the parties; and diſtinctly heard the enquiring rider ſay to his companion, " *If he'll let me ride her, I'll do him by G—d.*" " Nay, then I have an eye upon you," was a quotation that ſtruck me with the full force of the author. Luckily ſhielded with this confidence, I philoſophically made my appearance; when this *honeſt, worthy, immaculate* type of TURF INTEGRITY, made an apology for the liberty of troubling me, " but he underſtood I had a mare to run that day; that the oppoſite party had not uſed him well in ſome previous concerns; he wiſhed *to be revenged,* and with my permiſſion he would ride the mare GRATIS, in which he would exert his greateſt ability, and did not doubt but he ſhould be able to beat them *out of the world.*"

I was thankful to a degree of HUMILIATION for the liberality of his offer, perfectly conſcious of his kindneſs, and voluntary attention *to my intereſt*; but I was obſtinately determined to ſtand or fall by the effect of my own management, under

the

the additional difadvantage of a young and inexperienced rider.

Previous to the day of running, I had repeatedly and carefully inftructed my own lad in every minutiæ it became neceffary to have in conftant remembrance; naturally concluding to what an infinity of attacks and deep laid fchemes he would be eternally open previous to the hour of ftarting. I had particularly cautioned him, not to deliver *a weight* out of his pocket from the time of weighing to his return to the fcale after the race, upon any account whatever; not to *pull up* till he was confiderably paft the *winning poft*; nor to make even an effort to *difmount* till I led his horfe up *to the fcale.* All thefe very fortunately proved propitious precautions; for not one of the whole but was individually attacked, with a well fupported hope and unremitting expectation, of rendering us dupes to an eftablifhed courfe of villainy, - that it is to be regretted fo frequently fucceeds.

When juft going to ftart, a real friend, or rather *an honeft man,* who had that moment heard the fecret tranfpire in *a whifper,* came and

and told him they had weighed him, *ten stone four pounds*, placing *four pounds* in his pockets more than he was entitled to carry; advising him to ride up to the scale and insist upon being re-weighed; but adhering closely to my instructions, he refused to dismount, or relinquish a single weight, and absolutely won his match with *four pounds* more than he should have carried. Fifty yards before he reached the winning post, one of the party clamorously commanded him *to pull up*, saying, the other *" would never overtake him;"* the moment I had his horse by the bridle leading him to the scale, another vociferously enjoined him *" to get off and not distress the mare;"* either of which, not previously guarded against, but inadvertently complied with, must have inevitably lost the very considerable sum I had depending upon the event,

But to confirm beyond every shadow of doubt this horrid scene of deliberate villainy and deception; while the mare was rubbing down at a small distance from the course, after winning the race and receiving the stakes, a person came and made enquiry, whether *"* a jockey had not been with me that morn-

5   ing

ing early, making an offer to ride my mare,
GRATIS?" Upon my anfwering in the af-
firmative, he affured me I had a very narrow efcape; for " he had fat the preceding evening in an adjoining room, divided
only by a deal partition, and heard the entire
plan formed by the party concerned; that
if I confented to let him ride, my *mare was
to lofe*, and he was TO BE REWARDED."

However trifling or fuperfluous a recital
of thefe circumftances may appear to the
well informed and long experienced fportfman; they are no lefs neceffary with the juvenile adventurer, to eftablifh the exiftence
of facts, and expofe the various means of
almoft inexplicable *duplicity, invention,* and
impofition, by which the OPULENT, LIBE-
RAL, and INCONSIDERATE are fo frequently
reduced to a ftate of repentant deftruction.
Their introduction will confequently ferve to
render incontrovertible the proof of fuch practices; and to demonftrate the *folly* and *danger* of encountering fo great a complication of
deliberate villainy and fyftematick depredation, where there muft ever remain fo con-
fufed a profpect of extrication, with either

SUCCESS

SUCCESS or EMOLUMENT. Under the influence of fuch reflections as muft naturally arife from a knowledge of, and retrofpective allufion to, fuch incredible acts of villainy in conftant practice; every reader will be enabled to decide, whether it can poffibly tend to the promotion of his PLEASURE, INTEREST or SAFETY, to fufpend any part of his property by fuch doubtful dependencies. Confcious of no motive for the expofure of fuch abftrufe deception and complicated deftructive villainy, but an anxious contribution to the GENERAL GOOD; I am moft earneftly induced to hope the PURITY OF INTENTION may lay fome claim to the ftamp of public approbation, however deficient my flender abilities may have proved in the EXECUTION.

F I N I S.

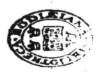

INDEX.

INDEX.

O.

P.

Q.

R.

Pectoral Detergent Balls, for Obftinate Coughs, } 9s.
   or Afthmatic and Thick Winded Horfes,
Fever Balls,   -   -   -   1s. 6d. each.
Balls for Loofenefs or Scouring   -   1s. 6d.
Balls for Strangury,   -   -   1s. 6d.
Balls for Flatulent Cholic, or Fret,   -   2s.
Balls for Inflammatory Cholic, or Gripes,   2s.
Bliftering Ointment, for Lamenefs, Spavins, } 3s. per pot.
   Splents, and Curbs,   -   -
Embrocation for Lamenefs, or Strains,   2s. 6d. per bottle.
Alterative Powders, for Cracks, Scratches, } 4s. per doz.
   Surfeit, Hidebound, Mange, or Greafe,

THE almoft unprecedented Portion of Public Favour that has fanctioned the Appearance of "THE GENTLEMAN'S STABLE DIRECTORY," and rendered the Publication of the *Eleventh Edition* unavoidably neceffary within the Space of *Three Years*, may be candidly confidered the incontrovertible Criterion of its Utility. The very flattering Marks of Approbation that have reached the Author, from fome of the moft diftinguifhed Characters, added to the preffing Perfuafions of others, equally high in the fporting World, have at length influenced him to render the Whole a complete Chain of Convenience to the Kingdom in general, by the perfonal Preparation of his moft efficacious Prefcriptions; a Plan fo evidently calculated to eradicate the very Foundation of EMPIRICAL IMPOSITION and MEDICAL ADULTERATION, that he cannot indulge a Doubt, but the Promotion of a general Good, will be honored with the Stamp of PUBLIC APPROBATION.

Mr. TAPLIN begs to add his moft grateful Acknowledgements to thofe Noblemen and Gentlemen, from whom he has received Permiffion of Reference for the Efficacy of his Medicines; and that every Plan may be adopted to render the Arrangement more acceptable, he wifhes it to be univerfally known, that Gentlemen refiding in remote Parts of the Country, who are defirous of keeping a fmall Affortment of Medicines for unexpected Emergencies, may always poffefs the Privilege of exchanging them for new Preparations at any Seafon of the Year, provided the characteriftic Seal has not been broken.

OF

O F

C. and G. KEARSLEY,

AT JOHNSON's HEAD, FLEET-STREET,

MAY BE HAD THE FOLLOWING

NEW PUBLICATIONS.

The HISTORY of FRANCE,
From the firft Eftablifhment of that Monarchy, brought down to, and
including
A complete NARRATIVE of the late REVOLUTION.
Res geftæ regumque ducumque, & triftia Bella.   HOR.
A new Edition, in Three Volumes, Octavo.
Price Eighteen Shillings in boards.
For Characters of the above Work, the Public are referred to the
Monthly, Analytical, Critical, European, and Englifh Reviews.

The HISTORY of ROME,
From the Foundation of the City by Romulus, to the Death of Marcus
Antoninus,
By the AUTHOR of the HISTORY of FRANCE.
Ret Romana, quæ ab exiguis profecta initiis, eo creverit, ut jam magni-
tudine laboret fua.   LIVY.
In Three Volumes, Octavo.
Price Eighteen Shillings in boards.

The HISTORY of SPAIN,
By the AUTHOR of the HISTORIES of FRANCE and ROME.
In Three Volumes, Octavo.
Price Eighteen Shillings in boards.

LETTERS to the Right Hon. EARL MANSFIELD, from ANDREW
STUART, Efq.
On the celebrated DOUGLAS CAUSE.
Price Seven Shillings and Six-pence, fewed.

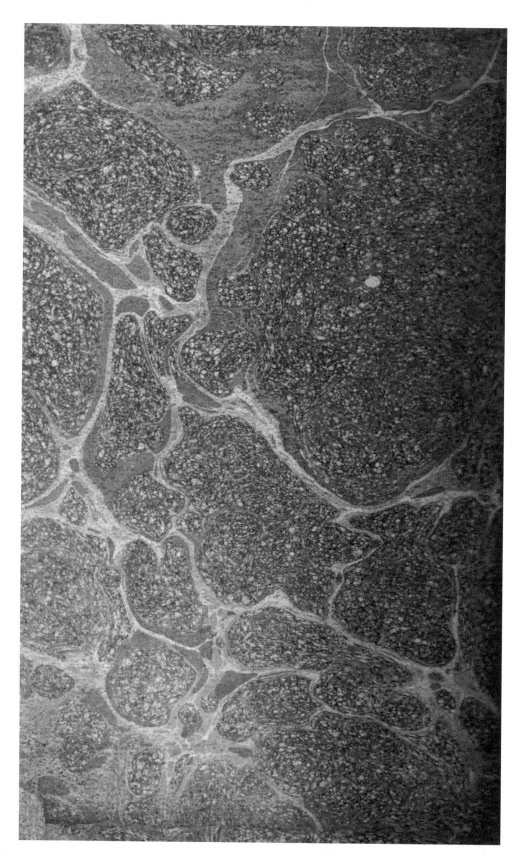

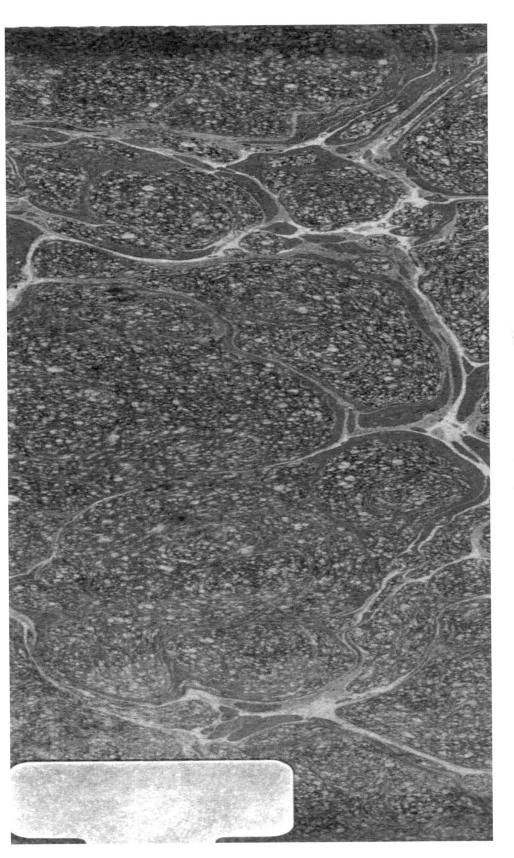

Check Out More Titles From HardPress Classics Series In this collection we are offering thousands of classic and hard to find books. This series spans a vast array of subjects – so you are bound to find something of interest to enjoy reading and learning about.

Subjects:
Architecture
Art
Biography & Autobiography
Body, Mind &Spirit
Children & Young Adult
Dramas
Education
Fiction
History
Language Arts & Disciplines
Law
Literary Collections
Music
Poetry
Psychology
Science
…and many more.

Visit us at www.hardpress.net

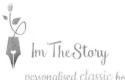
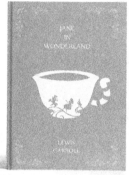